Writing for Canadian Health Professionals

Writing for Canadian Health Professionals

Lisa Salem-Wiseman
Humber College

Sobia Zaman
Humber College

NELSON / EDUCATION

NELSON / EDUCATION

Writing for Canadian Health Professionals

by Lisa Salem-Wiseman and Sobia Zaman

Vice President, Editorial Director:
Evelyn Veitch

Editor-in-Chief, Higher Education:
Anne Williams

Executive Editor:
Laura Macleod

Senior Marketing Manager:
Amanda Henry

Developmental Editor:
Theresa Fitzgerald

Photo Researcher:
Kristiina Paul

Permissions Coordinator:
Kristiina Paul

Content Production Manager:
Claire Horsnell

Production Service:
MPS Limited, a Macmillan Company

Copy Editor:
Dianne Fowlie

Proofreader:
Jennifer McIntyre

Indexer:
David Luljak

Production Coordinator:
Ferial Suleman

Design Director:
Ken Phipps

Managing Designer:
Franca Amore

Interior Design:
Peter Papayanakis

Cover Design:
Peter Papayanakis

Cover Image:
David Joel/Jupiter Images

Compositor:
MPS Limited, a Macmillan Company

Library and Archives Canada Cataloguing in Publication

Salem-Wiseman, Lisa
Writing for Canadian health professionals / Lisa Salem-Wiseman, Sobia Zaman.

Includes index.
ISBN 978-0-17-650148-8

1. Medical writing. I. Zaman, Sobia, 1969- II. Title.
R119.S35 2011   808'.06661
C2010-904872-5

ISBN 13: 978-0-17-650148-8
ISBN 10: 0-17-650148-7

Icon Image Credits: "Anecdotes" icon (health professional taking notes): © Ron Hohenhaus/Istock. "Try It Yourself" icon (notebook and pen): Photos.com. "COCOACAT" icon (coffee cup and saucer with smiling cat in latte): © Melissa Tee Photography/Flickr/Getty Images. "Canadian content" icon (maple leaf): Ydefinitel/Shutterstock. "Reflection" icon (thinking woman): Sami Sarkis Lifestyles / Alamy.

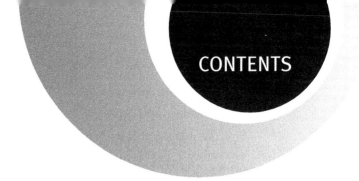

CONTENTS

CHAPTER 3: WRITING IN A PROFESSIONAL SETTING   75

CHAPTER 4: ETHICS IN HEALTH CARE: THE BASICS   97

CHAPTER 5: CREATIVE CONNECTIONS: HEALTH DISCUSSIONS AND CONTROVERSIES   113

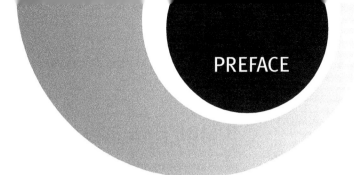

The idea for *Writing for Canadian Health Professionals* grew out of several frustrating and fruitless searches for a writing textbook for our pre-health science students. We both teach writing courses aimed at students interested in becoming paramedics, nurses, occupational therapist assistants, physiotherapist assistants, personal support workers, and pharmacy assistants. These are all fields in which poor written communication can have tragic consequences; therefore, it is essential that students in these programs learn to write accurately and effectively. Experience has taught us that these students learn communication skills best when their textbook incorporates health-related themes and content.

Unfortunately, although several colleges now offer courses specifically designed for students in the health sciences, there are very few writing textbooks designed specifically for the college and undergraduate health sciences student. We were looking for a textbook that (a) was Canadian, (b) was accessible to both the college and the university audience, (c) addressed the types of writing that students would be expected to produce in college and undergraduate university health sciences programs, (d) addressed the types of writing that graduates of these programs would be expected to produce in their workplaces, and (e) used examples from the real world of health care. When we were unable to find such a book, we decided to write it ourselves!

Writing for Canadian Health Professionals is the first of its kind in terms of student accessibility and Canadian content. It has been designed to help students in college and university health sciences programs as well as health professionals who wish to upgrade or review skills required to communicate effectively in writing. This book covers essential skills for any Canadian health sciences student or health care professional, including:

- conducting research using databases, search engines, and libraries
- documenting sources using APA format
- summarizing and analyzing written texts
- writing and formatting academic essays and reports
- writing effective resumés and cover letters
- communicating professionally by email
- writing narrative progress notes and structured progress notes
- understanding ethics and its importance in the health care workplace
- critically thinking about and expressing opinions on common and controversial health topics

In creating this text, we drew upon our experiences teaching writing to health sciences and pre-health sciences students, and we consulted colleagues, students, and health care professionals to ensure that the information and advice offered in this book is relevant, current, and practical.

INSIDE THIS BOOK

All chapters include:

- a list of **objectives**, so that students will clearly see what they can expect to have mastered by the end of the chapter
- a short **introduction**, explaining the relevance of the lessons to be covered
- **anecdotes** from health care professionals, chosen to illustrate the lessons in each chapter. These are indicated by the Anecdotes icon, featuring a health professional taking notes, as shown in the margin on the left.

- "try it yourself" **exercises** to give students a chance to practise the new skills that they have learned. This is indicated by the Notebook icon, shown on the left.

Some chapters include:

- an explanation of how students can use the **eight essential characteristics** of effective writing (outlined in Chapter One) to achieve success in the types of writing covered in the chapter. This is indicated by the COCOACAT icon, featuring a cocoa cup and a smiling cat, shown on the left (see page 7 for more on COCOACAT).
- provocative **articles, stories and poems** about important and controversial health issues. Canadian content is indicated by the Maple Leaf icon on the left.

- **discussion** questions that allow students to reflect on important health-related concerns and controversies. This is indicated by the Reflection icon, featuring a person deep in thought, on the left.
- **examples** from student assignments and/or professional documents

Chapter One shows why good writing is crucial in the health professions and provides a list of eight essential characteristics of effective writing for health professionals.

Chapter Two introduces students to common documents that they will be expected to produce in academic health sciences programs.

Chapter Three introduces students to common documents that they will be expected to produce in a professional context.

Chapter Four defines ethics, explores some of the ethical situations that health sciences students and health professionals might face, and provides excerpts from the codes of ethics for various professional organizations, including the Paramedic Association of Manitoba, the Canadian Physiotherapy Association, and the Canadian Nurses Association.

Chapter Five encourages students to think and write about important health issues and themes by exploring provocative health-related fiction and film.

We are both very excited by the publication of *Writing for Canadian Health Professionals,* particularly at the prospect of finally having an accessible, practical, and informative classroom resource that will help our students academically and professionally prepare for their future career in the health sciences field. As much of the book's content has already been "class-tested," we are confident that this resource will help you achieve your goals, both inside and outside of the classroom.

Happy teaching and learning!

Lisa Salem-Wiseman and Sobia Zaman

ACKNOWLEDGMENTS

The idea for this book was conceived while we were both teaching writing to pre-health students in Humber's General Arts and Science program, so the first and most important thanks go to our students, who encouraged us to write this book and who have been generous with their input and feedback over the last few years. Specific mention goes to contributors Erlinda Taruc, Deejay Gonzales, Winter Hill, Rachel Orsini, and Selina Tang. Gratitude is also due to our colleagues at Humber for their encouragement and enthusiasm—special thanks go to Judy Clarke, Colin Macrae, Patricia Morgan, Wendy Phillips, Mary Takacs, and the Humber College Career Centre.

Thanks also go to the Nelson Education higher education team for their dedication and effort: Laura Macleod, Amanda Henry, Franca Amore, Theresa Fitzgerald, Claire Horsnell, Dianne Fowlie, and Kristiina Paul.

We also greatly benefited from the feedback offered by those who reviewed both the proposal for this book and the early drafts, including Barbara Buetter, Niagara College, and Wanda Pierson, Langara College.

On a personal note, Lisa would like to acknowledge the support and patience of Jonathan and Rachel, as well as the expertise of her parents, both of whom have had successful careers as health professionals, and both of whom are excellent writers.

Sobia would like to dedicate this book to the memory of her sister-in-law, Janet Yorga, who lost her ferocious battle with cancer during the writing of this text and whose kindness and attitude will always continue to inspire. Sobia also wishes to acknowledge the special individuals in her life who encouraged and supported her involvement in this rewarding project.

WHAT YOU NEED TO KNOW ABOUT WRITING IN THE HEALTH SCIENCES

At the end of this chapter, you should be able to:

- understand why good writing skills are essential for a health sciences career
- apply the eight essential characteristics of effective writing in the health sciences
- complete relevant exercises that test your knowledge and application of the eight essential characteristics of good writing
- analyze and discuss real-life case studies in order to understand the serious consequences of documentation errors in health care

INTRODUCTION

More often than not, students interested in a health sciences career are disappointed when they see writing courses on their program timetables. College and university writing professors often encounter the following responses from their students: "I know how to write!"; "I don't need a writing course!"; "What does grammar have to do with saving lives?"; "This is a waste of time!" Judging by these fairly typical student reactions to English study, it appears that the student interested in paramedics just wants to "jump in" and start saving lives as opposed to attending to any deficiencies in spelling or grammar. Similarly, the nursing student becomes focused on what it takes to nurse others and would rather study blood pressure and medication administration than learn how to write clearly and concisely. Such common responses to English courses in the health care stream clearly demonstrate a lack of awareness concerning the important role writing plays in that field.

As you go through this chapter, you will discover the reasons why post-secondary health sciences programs make every effort to ensure that their graduates have good writing skills. While health sciences students may not find writing courses as "sexy" as anatomy or psychology, the following chapter outlines why these courses should be taken seriously and illustrates how they can have a tremendous impact, both academically and professionally.

This chapter begins by discussing why writing well in health care is a must, proceeds to illustrate the particular writing traits desired in the health care professions, and then presents, for discussion and analysis, real-life case scenarios that demonstrate the consequences of bad writing in health care.

SEVEN REASONS WHY WRITING IN THE HEALTH SCIENCES IS AN ESSENTIAL SKILL

Writing is a crucial skill in most professions and even more so in the busy and challenging environment of health care because of its potential impact on the physical and mental well-being of individuals. If you are planning to enter a health care field, what follows are seven good reasons why you must be able to write properly.

1) Your College or University Program Requires It

Unfortunately, success in a health care field cannot come without first meeting the academic demands of a postsecondary institution. And success in most academic programs depends on a student's ability to communicate his or her thoughts effectively. Whether an individual is pursuing a four-year university degree or a two-year college diploma, he or she must demonstrate some degree of writing proficiency in order to be successful in his or her academic training. In a Bachelor of Nursing program, for example, students are expected to show competence in various types of document writing including research reports, literature reviews, health promotion assignments, progress reports, and field reports. A student's inability to handle the writing demands of such tasks can lead to failure.

In addition to program-specific writing, health sciences students may find themselves in a position of having to take extra writing courses in order to upgrade their current skill level. These extra courses can vary greatly in content; some teach basic grammar concepts, while others offer practice with more complex and lengthier prose. Many postsecondary programs also require that health sciences students take electives or general education courses, many of which may be writing intensive.

It is also important to note that on the path to a rewarding health science career, a well-written, well-structured resumé and cover letter are essential. Individuals interested in working in the field of health sciences must, then, continue to demonstrate well-honed writing skills in order to effectively market themselves as competent professionals worthy of being hired.

2) Your Job Demands It

People are attracted to a career in the health sciences for a multitude of reasons, which may include a desire to help others, personal or familial experience with illness, or a desire to have a career as exciting as those portrayed in television dramas such as *ER* and *Grey's Anatomy*. Individuals lured into a health sciences career by the appeal and marketing of hospital-centred television dramas must, however, consider one of the least dramatic aspects of the job: the amount of writing involved. It has been estimated, for example, that physicians spend 90 percent of their jobs involved in some type of communication activity, a large part of which is writing (Terryberry, 2005). In addition to rounds and other responsibilities, nurses are required to complete assessment and progress notes and construct detailed patient care plans, as are many other health care providers. Health care professionals may also write research reports and educational materials, as well as contributing to professional journals. While many forms in health care facilities are designed to be user-friendly and efficient in their incorporation of checklists and flow charts, it is important to note that these documents are used in varying degrees at different institutions.

3) Communication Errors in the Workplace Translate into Incompetence

The Health Council of Canada, in their 2006 Annual Report, stated that "[T]he health of Canadians is being compromised by illegible handwriting and errors in the manual entry and processing of drug prescriptions" (p. 69), alluding to the role that poor penmanship and rushed data entry can play in sacrificing quality patient care. Despite the incorporation of computerized information management systems in many Canadian medical facilities, there are still some tasks that require handwriting, so neatnesss and legibility are paramount. This same report emphasizes that documentation systems in Canadian hospitals are in need of improvement in terms of efficiency, reliability, and accuracy (pp. 64–65).

Documentation errors in a medical facility occur for many different reasons and, ultimately, point to areas in need of improvement and change. In Canadian hospitals, inefficient documentation systems, lack of time to document comprehensively, the distractions of multi-tasking, and lack of proper education in the principles of professional written communication are often cited by health care workers as factors that inhibit their abilities to successfully handle important documentation-related tasks.

4) Others Look at What You Write

As in most occupations, health care professionals do not work independently; they are expected to work as members of a cooperative, effective, and efficient team. A patient in a hospital will likely have numerous attendants over the course of a hospital stay. In other words, there is more than one recorder of information as well as more than one reader of information. As all members of the health care team rely on the same notes for guidance, assessment, and treatment purposes, clarity and accuracy become the responsibility of each and every caregiver if quality patient care is to be maintained. It is clearly not feasible to hunt down previous caregivers, in a busy medical practice or hospital environment, for the purpose of seeking clarification on notes that should have been entered comprehensively and accurately in the first place. Rather, all documentation must be complete and precise at the time of recording so the patient in question will be treated effectively and efficiently by each and every member of the health care team that aids in his or her well-being.

5) Writing Well Protects You

If a patient dies under unusual circumstances or has unexpected complications, patient documentation becomes a key piece of evidence in determining the nature of complication or death as well as in constructing a reliable timeline in the event of a medical or criminal investigation. For the purposes of protection from accusations of wrongdoing, proper and accurate documentation is crucial; without comprehensive documentation, health care professionals set themselves, and their institutions, up for malpractice suits. Such suits drain time, energy, and resources of all involved and often end up damaging individual and institutional reputations.

In the sensitive area of health, individuals and families demand professional, honest, and reliable care from those trained to aid them. It is, for example, not uncommon for patients to attempt to sue health care practitioners or their institutions if they believe that their loved one was not treated or dealt with professionally, competently, or ethically. Indeed, such cases appear to be happening more frequently given the number of health-related malpractice suits.

One way in which health care providers can help protect themselves from false accusations and unreasonable malpractice suits is to ensure that anything they document is accurate and comprehensive. Written documentation is an important piece of evidence in the courtroom, where the spoken word has little weight in comparison to professional and detailed notes that effectively substantiate that an accused nurse or paramedic was not negligent. If there was no witness present at the time of an alleged incident with a patient, the written record of engagement with the patient is the only evidence chronicling the events leading up to an incident, complication, or death. Courts are impressed by accurate and complete notes, so health care practitioners must protect themselves and their institutions by leaving a trail of accurate and concise documentation. Additionally, the judicial process can be slow and tedious; archived medical records can be pulled up to be examined by coroners, police officers, and lawyers years after an incident. Human memory erodes over time, so legible, accurate, and comprehensive notes must compensate.

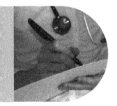

I've been a nurse for a long time and remember attending a professional development session, eons ago, where they showed a video clip of a lawyer questioning a nurse in some kind of malpractice case. The lawyer was ruthless! He had samples of the nurse's charting and blew it up on a HUGE

screen so that the judge and jury could see the errors it contained. The nurse didn't stand a chance; what defence is there for sloppy documentation? Her charts were almost illegible, with words scratched out. She also misused some standardized symbols. Even though I'm a nurse, I did not feel sorry for the woman on the videotape. If she looked incompetent and unprofessional, she brought that upon herself. The whole situation reminded me of how much our written documentation affects our reputation and credibility. This is serious stuff.

—RPN (hospital)

6) Writing Well Is a Tool for Advancement

It is rare that health care professionals will spend their entire career contributing to only one aspect of their profession. A bedside nurse, for example, may end up eventually in administration, in teaching, or in research. In administration, the ability to compile reports is often a necessity; similarly, in teaching, the preparation of accurate handouts and possible contributions to textbook material both require good writing skills. Good writing skills, therefore, become no less valuable but may, in fact, become even more essential in the event of promotion or change of duties within a particular health sector. An occupational therapist may decide, one day, to open her own business after several years of working for others. Without the proper writing skills to draft an effective proposal and business plan or the ability to effectively market herself, she faces a frustrating and perhaps failing endeavour.

The quality of written communication is an important measurement of professionalism in any workplace, including health care. Individuals with good writing skills are more likely to be viewed as competent professionals who are precise and detail-oriented in work tasks assigned to them. Such individuals are also often considered for promotions and other career-enhancing projects.

7) Your Patients Deserve the Absolute Best

Without a doubt, the most important reason for the emphasis on good writing skills in health care is that comprehensive and accurate documentation is essential for high-quality patient care. While there is much to debate in the complicated world of health care, it is very difficult to dispute that the primary role of the health care professional is to preserve the health and well-being of the patient; this goal, however, cannot be accomplished if documentation on that patient is fragmented, sloppy, or non-existent. Errors in care and treatment abound if, along the way, caregivers pay sloppy attention to detail, or fail to record crucial and relevant details such as a patient's allergies to or side effects from medications. If a patient's written medical history is mishandled, how can that patient receive accurate and responsible care? The course of a patient's treatment, the effect of that treatment, and any complications, must all

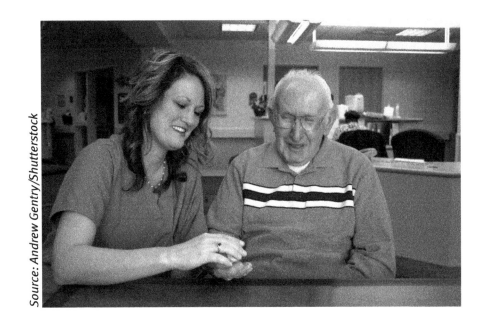

be recorded accurately in order to maintain high quality care—the ultimate goal of any health care provider.

CHARACTERISTICS OF WRITING FOR THE HEALTH SCIENCES

Now that we have established why writing well is important to the health professions, this section will focus on what exactly "writing well" means in the health context.

Every academic discipline has its own set of expectations for good writing, and the health sciences are no different. The elegant, imaginative, expressive style of writing that earned you an A in your high school or college literature class will not earn you the same mark in NRS 101: Nursing as a Profession or PSYC 121: Applied Psychology 1. You will be expected to produce assignments that are **clear, objective, concise, organized, accurate, correct, audience-appropriate,** and **thorough.**

Furthermore, once you graduate and are working in the health care industry, you will be expected to communicate in a clear, objective, concise, organized, accurate, correct, audience-appropriate, and thorough manner . . . and all while under extreme pressure in a fast-paced, stressful environment that is full of distractions!

Because health care workers often work in shifts, their coworkers need to be able to pick up their notes and understand exactly what is going on with a patient. Effective documentation is crucial to good patient care.

In order to help you become an effective communicator, we will introduce you to the eight qualities of health care communication that have been consistently identified as most important by qualified health care professionals. Whether you are writing a lab report for chemistry class, a research report on the Canadian health care system, an incident report, or notes on a patient's chart, these eight principles will help ensure that your communication is effective.

All you need to remember is:

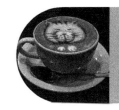

COCOA CAT

C	clear
O	objective
C	concise
O	organized
A	accurate
C	correct
A	audience-appropriate
T	thorough

C is for CLEAR

A common complaint of many health professionals is that much of the written communication they see in the workplace is unclear or vague and contains confusing wording.

Communication in the world of health care needs to be clear and unambiguous for the following reasons:

- Many health care workplaces are collaborative environments; therefore, others should be able to pick up a health care worker's notes and understand exactly what is going on with a patient.
- A misunderstood instruction can lead to serious or even fatal consequences.
- Documentation can be subpoenaed, so each piece needs to be able to stand on its own as a legal record.

Tips for Improving Clarity

1. When given a choice between a familiar term and an obscure term, the more familiar term is preferable, as long as the meaning stays the same. When writing for a general audience, define any technical terms that are specific to your profession.

2. Read over what you have written, asking yourself whether your intended meaning is obvious to the reader.

Remember: Bigger Isn't Always Better!

Sometimes an attempt to use "big words" backfires. If your reader does not understand what you are trying to say, your writing will not be effective.

TRY IT YOURSELF

Can you spot the unintentional blooper in each of the following real-life examples of nurses' writing? Using the space provided, correct each sentence to make its meaning clearer.

1. "Patient is awake and alert with many visitors in bed."

2. "Patient may shower with assistants."

3. "The resident came in from the garden and threw a dog at the television."

4. "Patient became ill after eating too many turtles while at the zoo."

5. "The nurse delivered the baby, cut and clamped the cord, and handed it to the paediatrician."

Source: Courtesy of Doctors Lounge: www.doctorslounge.com

O is for OBJECTIVE

Scientific writing must be objective, that is, free of personal assumptions, biases, feelings, or opinions. There are a few reasons for this:

- Results of tests or experiments will only be considered valid if another professional would be able to produce the same results. Therefore, the focus is on the work, not the worker.
- Notes and charts can be made public; therefore, judgments such as "the patient was whining," "the wound is giving off a disgusting odour," or "this patient is a nightmare" are inappropriate.
- Personal impressions are subjective, that is, dependent on a person's moods, opinions, attitudes, and beliefs. Such impressions communicate very little real information. If a person is described as "old," is he or she 45? 60? 95? Is a "hot" day 20 degrees Celsius? 30? 40?

Tips for Achieving an Objective Tone

1. Avoid starting sentences with "I" or "we": this pulls focus away from the scientific topic at hand.

2. Avoid using "I think" or "we believe." Everything you say should follow from logic, not from personal bias or subjectivity. Never use emotive words (such as feel, believe, or think) or words that imply judgment (such as seems, appears, or looks like).

3. Stick to what can be observed; don't "fill in the blanks" by making assumptions. If a patient stumbles when walking into a clinic and appears disoriented and confused while giving her history, do not record that "the patient was drunk." Record the behaviour, but don't guess at the cause, even if it seems to be obvious.

4. Avoid making judgments based on data. Record the data; don't interpret it.

TRY IT YOURSELF

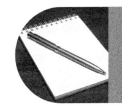

Here are a student's observations of an experiment in which a mouse in a maze was given two pathways to choose from, only one of which led to food. Underline all the SUBJECTIVE elements in this paragraph. Now, rewrite it as an OBJECTIVE, facts-only scientific description.

> *The little grey mouse carefully peered down each pathway. Finally, after thinking about it for a while, it decided to venture down the path on the right. The mouse started tentatively down that pathway, but it stopped, confused, when it failed to find any food. It turned around and went back to the start. I think the mouse must have been hungry, because it rushed down the pathway on the left and greedily gobbled up all of its food.*

C is for CONCISE

Health care professionals have to convey large amounts of information quickly, and in small spaces on forms and charts. It is important to be direct, avoid repetition and irrelevant information, and summarize data whenever possible.

Tips for Making Writing Concise

1. Avoid wordy phrases.

    "at this point in time" can be reworded as "now"

    "at a later date" can be reworded as "later"

2. Cut meaningless words or phrases.

Phrases such as the following add no meaning to your writing:

"all things considered"

"for all intents and purposes"

"as far as I'm concerned"

"in my opinion"

3. Avoid redundant or repetitive phrases:

"8 a.m. in the morning" can be changed to "8 a.m."

"fewer in number" can be changed to "fewer"

4. Combine sentences to reduce length.

Janet is studying. She is tired. She is preparing for her anatomy exam. It is her last exam.

Although Janet is tired, she is studying for her last exam, which is anatomy.

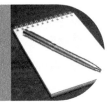

TRY IT YOURSELF

Rewrite the following sentences to eliminate repetition, irrelevant information, and empty words and phrases.

1. The accident occurred at 2 p.m. in the afternoon.

2. In this day and age, nursing is a popular career choice for men as well as women.

3. Eva's little brother was eating popcorn. A piece became stuck in his throat. He couldn't breathe. He was turning blue. Eva performed the Heimlich manoeuvre. The popcorn flew across the room. He gasped, coughed, and began breathing normally.

4. In the clinic, staff attend to critically ill patients who are very sick.

5. Due to the fact that the flu can be fatal, it is important for people 65 years of age or older to have a flu shot.

O is for ORGANIZED

For communication in the health professions to be effective, it needs to be organized in a logical manner that makes it easy to understand.

Tips for Improving Organization

1. State your main point clearly and near the beginning of your piece of writing.

2. Put the most important information first.

3. Make a statement or claim first, and then back it up with any details or examples.

4. When relating an incident, describe the events in the order in which they occurred (chronological order).

5. Use transitional words ("first," "next," "finally," "after," "therefore") and phrases ("as a result," "before beginning,") to connect ideas.

6. Use cues such as headings, topic sentences, transition words, lists, and graphics.

TRY IT YOURSELF

Rearrange the sentences in the following paragraph in a more logical order, adding transitional words and phrases when needed. You may combine sentences and/or omit words.

> *Dr. James Young, at St. Jude's hospital, examined me and told me that my left shoulder was dislocated. At 9:00 a.m. that morning, the store manager, Rose Daniels, asked me to hang a large plastic skeleton over the customer service desk. When I got to work that morning she had asked me to get the ladder from the storeroom. I leaned too far to the left and lost my balance. I climbed to the top rung and attempted to hang the skeleton, but I couldn't reach the hook on the ceiling. I landed on my left shoulder and couldn't move. I screamed in pain and Ms. Daniels called the paramedics. On Tuesday, October 23, I was injured when I fell off a ladder while hanging Halloween decorations in my workplace, David's Books.*

A is for ACCURATE

Accuracy is extremely important in scientific writing. An accurate description of the location of pain or the size of a wound or the amount of a substance to be administered could be vital.

Tips for Improving Accuracy

1. Pay attention to word choice and make sure that you are using the correct word. Know the terminology associated with the subject.

2. Include all essential information, including measurements and quantities.

3. Use proper names for people, places, and medications.

4. Avoid vague terms like "good" and "worse" and qualifiers such as "very" or "really." Give specific information.

What essential information is missing from the following paragraph? Edit the paragraph to make it more accurate. You will need to be creative and make up details.

Angela Jones arrived at the clinic early in the morning with her baby daughter, Maria. The child had a high fever and a bad cough. Ms. Jones told the receptionist that Maria had started coughing a few days ago and that the cough had gotten worse. After some time in the waiting room, Maria was taken to see a doctor, who prescribed some medicine.

C is for CORRECT

The first question that students ask upon receiving an assignment is usually "Does spelling count?" The answer should always be "Yes." One problem frequently cited by nurse managers, doctors, and other health professionals is basic errors in spelling, punctuation, and grammar. Such errors reflect poorly upon the writer, and are often assumed to be a sign of a more general carelessness or lack of attention to detail; in the health professions, such carelessness can—quite literally—be fatal. Misspelled drug names, misplaced decimals, grammatical errors, or misused words could have serious consequences.

Tips for Correcting Errors

If you are writing on a computer, use the spelling check software, but do not rely on it too much. In addition, try the following:

1. Use a dictionary when you write.

2. Familiarize yourself with commonly confused words.

3. Proofread everything you have written.

4. Use correct grammar. Your word processor's grammar checker can help you to identify errors, but you should keep a grammar handbook nearby to ensure that you know how to correct them.

5. Read carefully, thinking about the logic of what you have written.

Check and double-check the spelling of all proper nouns, including people's names, locations, addresses, procedures, equipment, and medications. Some **commonly confused words** include the following:

- ACCEPT: to receive
  EXCEPT: to take or leave out; excluding

  I will **accept** all the applications **except** for yours.

- AFFECT: to influence (verb)
  EFFECT: a result (noun)

The **effect** of sun exposure is premature aging of the skin.

Too much exposure to sun has **affected** her appearance.

- A LOT: many
  ALOT: no such word

We saw **a lot** of patients this morning.

- ALL RIGHT: satisfactory
  ALRIGHT: disputed variant of "all right" not yet widely accepted as correct

Joanne was feeling **all right** until she saw her midterm grade.

- ITS: of or belonging to it
  IT'S: a contraction of "it is"

It's not a good sign that your dog keeps scratching **its** ears.

- LAY: to put down; to place somewhere
  LIE: to be in a horizontal position

Lay the book on the table before you **lie** down for a nap.

- LOSE: to misplace; to not win (v.)
  LOOSE: not tight (adj./adv.)

The clasp on my necklace is **loose**; I'm afraid I might **lose** it.

- PRINCIPAL: main or most important (adj.); a person who has authority (n.)
  PRINCIPLE: a general or fundamental truth

His **principal** concern was the cost of the project.

The textbook covers the basic **principles** of genetics.

- THAN: used with comparisons
  THEN: at that time; next

I'm doing better in math **than** I am in chemistry.

I'll study chemistry first, and **then** I'll review my math notes.

- THEIR: belonging to them
  THERE: indicates location
  THEY'RE: contraction of "they are"

They're moving **their** offices to that building over **there**.

Find the errors in the following sentences.

1. Franklin was thrilled when he was excepted into the paramedicine program.

2. Take two Aspirins and lay down for an hour.

3. I think I did alright on the exam.

4. What are the common side affects of that medication?

5. Lupus is sometimes misdiagnosed because it's symptoms are often mistaken for the symptoms of other diseases.

A is for AUDIENCE-APPROPRIATE

Consider the needs of your audience. An audience of medical professionals will be familiar with specialized terminology and will expect and need information that the general public will not.

Tips for Determining the Needs of Your Audience

Ask yourself the following questions:

1. Who are my readers? (Consider such things as age, gender, occupation, economic/educational background, and political or religious beliefs.)

2. Why will they be reading this document?

3. What do they need to know?

4. What do they already know? What do I need to tell them?

5. How specialized should my language be? How formal or informal? Do I need to define any terms?

6. Will they read every word or scan for key information? How can I help ensure that my message is received?

The following passage is taken from the report of an emergency room physician after performing a stump appendectomy on a 34-year-old woman. The audience is the patient's family doctor. Rewrite the passage for a non-specialized audience, for example, the patient's husband.

The patient was brought to the emergency room by ambulance at 0300 hours, August 11, 2007, for investigation of severe abdominal pains, nausea, and vomiting. Physical examination revealed a soft mass in the lower quadrant of the abdomen. Blood examination showed leukocytosis (white blood cell count 11,600/mm3) and an elevated C reactive protein (CRP) level (4.7 mg/dl). Computed tomography (CT) and ultrasonography of the abdomen showed an intraluminal mass. A preoperative diagnosis of stump appendicitis was made on the basis of the CT study. Stump appendicitis is a rare clinicopathologic entity characterized by inflammation of the appendiceal remnant after incomplete appendectomy.

T is for THOROUGH

In the health professions, it is important that all communication be thorough and complete to ensure the best possible care. Many patient notes omit essential information—instead of writing that a patient walked 30 feet, the health care worker should include that the patient needed a walker and was displaying shortness of breath. In addition, many insurance claims do not get paid because information is missing from medical notes. Finally, incomplete documentation could result in a negligence lawsuit; there is a saying in the health professions: "If it wasn't documented, then, legally, it wasn't done."

Tips for Making Your Writing Thorough

1. Make a checklist of all the information that your reader needs to know.

2. Include all measurements and specifications. Be specific.

3. Include all relevant proper names—of people, places, medications, etc.

4. Proofread carefully, looking for missed steps or gaps in logic or information.

5. Ask yourself: if you were someone unfamiliar with the information being communicated, would you have any questions?

TRY IT YOURSELF

The following is an excerpt from a letter to an insurance company, asking for compensation. It is missing crucial information. Rewrite the paragraph, adding any missing details that you consider to be important.

The other week, while driving along Locust Street, I was hit by another car. My rear bumper was badly dented. The driver of the other vehicle was very apologetic and told me that she would take me to the hospital. I have severe whiplash and will have to stay home from work for a while.

The following two pieces of writing illustrate the difference between a personal narrative and an objective account that corresponds with the eight principles discussed above. The first piece (Box 1.1) is a short personal essay in which a student recounts the events surrounding her sister's injury; in the second piece (Box 1.2), the student has revised her account as an INCIDENT REPORT to make it clear, objective, concise, organized, accurate, correct, audience-appropriate, and thorough.

BOX 1.1   Personal Narrative

When my sister Gillian was about four years old, she smacked her head on the stairs to our basement and cut her eyebrow open. Gillian, my brother, and I were all in the basement watching TV when my mother called us up for lunch. We all bounded up the steps. My brother and I reached the top before my sister because she wasn't as fast as us, so we pushed her out of the way and went to the kitchen. She decided to go up the stairs on her hands and feet like a dog; one of her hands missed a step and she slipped off the stair and smashed her face onto the concrete stairs. She had hit the stair pretty hard, so she was dizzy and fell down the five or six steps she had already climbed. My mom heard her crying and ran to help her. When my mom saw that the stairs were covered in blood, she panicked. The gash in Gillian's head was so deep that we could see her skull. At the hospital, the doctor stitched her up and said that she was lucky because she could have fractured her skull. She had a lot of bruising on her face but was otherwise fine. She got some kind of anti-inflammatory pills to help with the pain and took a week off school.

BOX 1.2   Objective Account

TO: Greg Kelley, Principal of Queen of Heaven Elementary School

FROM: Rachel Orsini, Sibling/Witness

DATE: September 21, 2007

SUBJECT: Report of incident (20/09/2007) in which Gillian Orsini was injured.

Gillian Orsini's right eyebrow was injured on September 20, 2007, in an accident that occurred at 1093 Gardner Avenue in Mississauga. She was taken to the Trillium Health Centre, where her right eyebrow was stitched and bandaged. She will be unable to attend school for one week.

The accident occurred at approximately 12:30 p.m., while walking up a flight of stairs. Gillian was walking in the basement of 1093 Gardner Avenue, when she was called to lunch. Gillian then proceeded to climb up the stairs.

As Gillian went up the stairs, she slipped and fell onto the concrete steps, landing on the right side of her face. She then fell down the stairs and landed at the base of the steps.

Immediately after Gillian fell, Andrea Orsini, Gillian's mother, came to her aid. Gillian was bleeding profusely from a wound above her right eye. Mrs. Orsini then proceeded to take Gillian to the Trillium Health Centre, where Gillian's right eyebrow was stitched and bandaged.

According to Dr. K. Smith, Gillian sustained a laceration on her right eyebrow, one-half inch deep, as well as severe facial bruising to the right side of her face. No other injuries were reported.

Dr. K. Smith prescribed Tylenol 3, to help ease Gillian's discomfort. This medication will make her very drowsy. Therefore, for the duration that Gillian will be on the medication, she will not be able to attend school. Dr. K. Smith said that she may return after one week.

Exercise

1. Write a subjective, first-person account of an incident that you either experienced or witnessed. You should use the first person ("I") and include your observations, thoughts, and feelings about the experience.

   Exchange it with a partner, and read each other's accounts, looking for **clarity, objectivity, conciseness, organization, accuracy, correctness, audience-appropriateness,** and **thoroughness.** Highlight or underline the words and passages that need to be changed.

   Then, return each other's papers and edit your own, transforming it into a **clear, objective, concise, organized, accurate, correct, audience-appropriate,** and **thorough** account of the incident.

THE CONSEQUENCES OF POOR DOCUMENTATION: REAL-LIFE CASE STUDIES

You have now learned why writing well in health care is important as well as what writing well in health care means. The following two real-life case studies (Box 1.3 and Box 1.4) demonstrate the devastating consequences that can arise from negligent documentation in a health care environment and synthesize everything you have learned so far about the importance of accurate and comprehensive documentation. Work in pairs or groups to discuss the questions that follow each case.

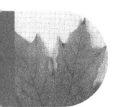

BOX 1.3

"A grief without end; Hospital apologizes to 11-year-old's family for the errors that killed her"

"Senior staff at Hamilton Health Sciences have accepted responsibility for the death of 11-year-old Claire Lewis and have offered their "profound apologies" to the girl's family.

Apologizing and accepting responsibility is highly unusual for a hospital.

However, parents John and Brenda Lewis say the hospital's actions mean little. They won't find solace until the doctors, residents, and nurses, whose series of egregious errors led to their daughter's death, come forward and apologize.

"It's like having your child killed by a drunk driver, and the CEO of the insurance company apologizes on behalf of the client. It's ludicrous, it's self-important and it's just silly," said John Lewis.

In the summer of 2001, a neurosurgeon discovered a benign tumor near the base of her brain.

On Oct. 12 of that year, she underwent surgery to remove the tumor at Hamilton General Hospital. After a successful 8 1/2-hour operation, Claire was transferred to McMaster University Medical Centre's pediatric intensive care unit to recover.

"She was a perfectly beautiful child. Well on her way to recovery," John Lewis, himself a nurse, said.

A long line of errors and poor decisions over the next 46 hours killed Claire.

The first mistake happened when doctors transferred her between hospitals.

Her medical records did not go with her.

As a result, staff at MUMC didn't know what fluids Claire had received or in what quantities. Then John and Brenda Lewis's daughter was misdiagnosed with diabetes insipidus, a common post-operative complication characterized by excessive fluid loss through the urine. The staff repeatedly gave her a drug called DDAVP so she would retain fluids, not knowing the last thing Claire needed was to retain fluid.

Then, a transcription of the DDAVP order left out the words "call endocrinology," and the on-duty endocrinologist was not consulted.

As pressure built in Claire's cranium, John watched in horror as his daughter began shaking. Her tremors escalated into a full-blown three-minute seizure. Staff adjusted her sodium levels and continued to give her fluids for diabetes insipidus, also known as water diabetes, which she didn't have.

By noon on Oct. 14, Claire was awake, talking, eating and telling her 14-year-old sister, Jesse, that she loved her. The family left her alone for part of the afternoon and returned around 6:20 p.m. They found Claire "flat as a pancake," unconscious and non-responsive.

Jesse was so scared she ran from the hospital room. John went to the nursing station and demanded that a doctor examine Claire immediately. A resident arrived and examined the girl, but didn't take any action.

The hospital's own review concludes that if he had acted, Claire would be alive.

Claire's breathing slowed while John Lewis begged the nurse for help. When her breathing stopped, a senior physician finally arrived but it was too late. Claire's brain stem was crushed by excessive fluid. She was brain dead.

That John Lewis even knew his daughter's death was the result of errors and negligence can only be attributed to his training as a nurse and his knowledge of the medical system. It frightens him to think of the number of parents who never find out their children died from medical mistakes.

Four months passed after the girl's death before the hospital agreed to meet with her parents. Six months passed before the staff investigated, took responsibility and apologized. The family says the apology didn't come willingly and it wouldn't have come without their push.

HHS Chief of Staff Dr. Andrew McCallum, who co-authored the six-page apology with chief nursing officer Margaret Keatings and chief executive Murray Martin, said the apology is part of a new culture of disclosure in health care.

"Clearly it didn't happen in an ideal way. We regret that very much. It took too long and we acknowledge that," McCallum said.

"We didn't find a single person or a single event that led to this. We found a series of events and occurrences, slips, lapses, errors in judgment that led to this tragic outcome," he said. The hospital has since taken many steps to ensure that the same errors can't happen again, including changing its systems and re-educating its staff.

"It's been devastating for the institution. The people involved are terribly upset. We feel terribly for the loss the family has suffered. We offered our profound apologies. Claire's death could have been avoided," he said.

Paul Harte, the Lewis family's lawyer, said he believes the apology is the result of both his clients' badgering and a changing health-care culture. More amazing, he says, is that the family received an apology at all.

"All I do is sue doctors and nurses," said Harte, who has been a medical malpractice specialist for almost nine years. "I've never had occasion to see a hospital admit liability. The hospital should be lauded for admitting responsibility."

Lawyers for Hamilton Health Sciences and the Lewis family are close to reaching a settlement.

Sitting by the Christmas tree, the heavy scent of cooked vegetables and incense in the air, John Lewis acknowledged that his family may seem composed on the surface.

The reality is that the Lewis family's pain is excruciatingly potent 14 months after Claire's death. John says no one can understand the depth and power of their grief but those who have experienced the loss of a child themselves.

"We get out of bed in the morning, put a foot in front of the other, keep breathing and get through the day. Not a day goes by that there's not tears in this house."

He retells the story of Claire's death and the hospital's response with a simmering fury. Short breaks and deep breaths are necessary to keep from boiling over.

"Not one of (the staff members whose errors claimed Claire's life) has stepped forward and said, I am responsible and accountable for this. I want an acknowledgement of my child's life and my child's death and of my pain and suffering. I want them to look at me and say, 'I'm sorry sir, it will never happen again.'"

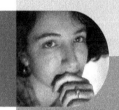

Discussion Questions:

1. What happened to Claire Lewis?

2. What factors led up to Claire's death?

3. What role did poor documentation or poor record-keeping play in Claire's death?

4. Could Claire's death have been prevented? If so, how?

5. How did the hospital respond to the situation?

6. How did the family respond to the situation?

7. Why is the family's lawyer surprised by the hospital's apology?

8. Does the family accept the hospital's apology? Why or why not?

9. Does anything in this story shock or surprise you?

10. What does this case teach us about documentation in health care?

BOX 1.4

"Another baby is given morphine by mistake: Boy survives after same hospital that gave infant fatal overdose makes second drug error"

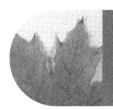

"A second baby has been mistakenly injected with morphine at Brampton's Peel Memorial Hospital.

A doctor at the hospital gave 9-month-old Juliano Pariselli the drug instead of codeine in an operating room, just before the baby underwent surgery to repair a hernia Feb. 15. Juliano survived, but his parents are worried about future health problems the error may cause.

It's the second time in eight months a child has received morphine by mistake at the hospital. Two morphine injections given mistakenly by a pediatric nurse killed 11-month-old Trevor Landry last June 24.

An inquest followed and the hospital said it had implemented procedures to prevent such medication errors from happening again.

"I was horrified," said Sabina Pariselli, who was by her son's crib last week when a nurse noticed the baby in distress and needing oxygen. "I knew something wasn't right. . . . I immediately thought of the Landrys."

The 26-year-old mother said she didn't know what had occurred, but was later told her son had been given the wrong drug.

Toronto lawyer Harry McMurtry, who represents Sabina Pariselli and her husband Bruno, said documents obtained from the hospital indicate Juliano was given three milligrams of morphine.

A document prepared by Dr. Gail Hirano said Juliano was supposed to receive 12 milligrams of codeine before surgery.

The mistake was noted at noon by Hirano on the doctor's orders and progress report.

"Patient received morphine . . . instead of codeine at 08:30," Hirano's handwritten note reads. "Explained to mother that medication error occurred and that Juliano would be observed in PACU (pediatric acute care unit) until . . . effects of morphine have passed."

Sabina said she was not immediately told how much morphine Juliano had been given and there was no indication on the baby's medical chart.

She said she repeatedly checked the chart, but there was never any indication of the dose administered. It wasn't until she and her husband were able to obtain copies of their son's records from the hospital a couple of days later that they saw a notation that Juliano had been given three milligrams of morphine.

According to the Canadian doctors' pharmaceutical bible, the Compendium of Pharmaceuticals and Specialties, three milligrams of morphine is equivalent to 36 milligrams of codeine. An appropriate dose of morphine for a baby of Juliano's weight would be between 0.9 milligrams and 1.8 milligrams, the compendium says.

Dr. Tom Dickson, the hospital's chief of medical staff, said he couldn't legally discuss Juliano's case because his parents hadn't given him permission to disclose any confidential patient information. He suggested drug and medication errors are a fact of life in hospitals around the world.

"It's a universal problem and the rate of drug error will never be reduced to zero.

"It's not a practical possibility, but we all aim to try to reduce the potential for error."

Using the media is not the way to deal with errors involving drugs and drawing parallels between recommendations from the Landry inquest and the most current case is inappropriate and not constructive, he said.

"The proper way of dealing with these is through careful study of why mistakes are made and how they are made and deal with the processes that make them."

A hospital spokesperson said Hirano would not comment.

The Parisellis said they are not satisfied the hospital records accurately reflect how much morphine Juliano was given.

Sabina said the copy of the form used to document the amount of narcotic administered and discarded was not included in documents provided to them by the hospital.

McMurtry, the father of three young children, said the public needs to be made aware.

"We're very unhappy with the state of affairs. The bottom line is we don't want another Landry case.

"There's no question the wrong medication was administered. . . . We want an explanation for why this occurred. We want answers."

Bruno Pariselli, 33, said he and his wife think about Trevor Landry every day and worry about what could have happened to Juliano.

"I don't know if I could exist without my son," he said.

Sabina said she couldn't live with herself if they didn't pursue this and another child died.

She said she's never experienced anything like the panic she felt when she realized her baby had been given the wrong medication.

"I would have absolutely no reason to live if I didn't have him," she said.

"He's a ham. He's a vibrant, happy kid. I got a little bit of a dose of what the Landrys felt. A little dose and I couldn't even bear that."

Juliano received the incorrect medication the same week a coroner's jury looking into Trevor's death was considering recommendations to prevent those kinds of errors from happening again.

During 22 days of testimony, the jury learned that Trevor, son of Cathy and Michael Landry of South Porcupine in the Timmins area, died after inadvertently being given two lethal doses of morphine by a nurse at the Brampton hospital.

Nurse Heather Leach incorrectly transcribed a doctor's written orders and mistakenly gave the child morphine.

Dickson said public attention about drug errors in hospitals generates fear about the kind of care people might receive in the health care system.

"We choose to take a constructive approach to errors as opposed to one that . . . may even trivialize what is really a very significant problem in the health care industry," he said.

Dickson said when a physician error occurs, there is a process at Peel Memorial Hospital that involves full disclosure to the family and an explanation of the events.

There is also a full investigation surrounding any events, including a review of procedures to determine if any changes are needed, he said.

There are different procedures in an operating room where a physician in the course of giving an anesthetic will administer many different and very potent drugs, he said.

"Doctors make those judgment calls, calculate their own dosages, administer the drugs, then wake the patients up and assume full responsibility for that procedure.

"It's not a situation like on a ward where individuals write an order, someone else transcribes it, someone else follows the order and someone else may administer the order," he said.

"In an operating room it is one individual who in fact writes the order, gets the drug, delivers the drug, documents from beginning to end. So it's an entirely different situation."

It's the third time Juliano has undergone surgery at the hospital after being born with a dislocated hip.

Sabina said because her son has been in hospital so often she is familiar with how he quickly recovers from anesthetics.

When Juliano was still in a deep sleep, nine hours after surgery, Sabina asked a nurse to call a pediatrician.

"The nurse wouldn't get a pediatrician, so I got really upset with her and said I knew about the Landry story and didn't want the same thing to happen to my son," she said.

Within minutes, two doctors were checking on Juliano's condition.

"We lost faith in the whole health care system," Sabina said.

Juliano was kept in hospital overnight and discharged the next day. When the baby developed a high fever later in the day, his parents took him to York Central Hospital.

"We didn't trust Peel," said Bruno, who had also undergone surgery at the same hospital that day.

"If they come in with a glass of water I'll ask what they are doing," he said. "It's scary that you have to do that."

Source: Tracy Huffman and Cal Millar, "Another baby is given morphine by mistake: Boy survives after same hospital that gave infant fatal overdose make a second drug error." Toronto Star, Feb. 26, 1999. Reprinted with permission—Torstar Syndication Services.

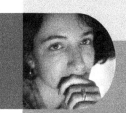

Discussion Questions:

1. What happened to Juliano Pariselli?

2. What role did documentation errors and omissions play in this case?

3. Were any of these errors preventable? If so, how?

4. How did the hospital respond to the situation?

5. How did the family respond to the situation?

6. While Juliano survived, his parents are still worried. Why?

7. What happened at the same hospital just eight months before?

8. What long-term effects has this situation had on the Pariselli family?

9. Did anything about this case shock or surprise you? If so, what?

10. What does this case teach us about proper record-keeping in hospitals?

CHAPTER 2

WRITING IN AN ACADEMIC SETTING

At the end of this chapter, you should be able to:

- recognize and produce various types of documents commonly assigned in health sciences programs
- write effective academic documents, including summaries, critical analyses, academic essays, and academic reports
- distinguish between paraphrasing and plagiarism and understand why the latter must be avoided
- conduct academic research, including determining the credibility of sources
- prepare a formal academic essay or report according to APA specifications
- correctly document sources using APA style guidelines

INTRODUCTION

As employers in the health professions are realizing the importance of writing well, more college and university programs are placing a greater emphasis on writing. Many students enter their programs unprepared for the types of academic documents they will have to produce and are unfamiliar with the skills of summarizing, analyzing, persuading, researching, incorporating sources into their writing, or documenting sources. In the following chapter, you will learn tips for approaching some of the typical writing assignments in health-related programs.

THE SUMMARY

In your college or university health program, you may be asked to write a summary of an article, chapter, or book.

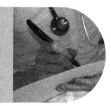

One of the most difficult things I had to do as a first-year nursing student was write an annotated bibliography for a research paper. I knew how to prepare a list of references in APA format, but I had no idea how to summarize an entire book or academic article in a short paragraph. It took me many tries to get the summaries short enough; I think I spent more time writing the summaries than I did writing the actual paper!

Nursing student, Vancouver, BC

A summary is a short restatement of the main idea and major points of a piece of writing. (See Box 2.1 and Box 2.2, pp. 27–29.) The length of a summary depends on the length of the original text; a summary of a book may be a page or two long, while a summary of a short article may only be a paragraph in length. The summary should not exceed one-third of the length of the original document.

The goal of writing a summary is to communicate the central argument, purpose, structure, main ideas, and supporting points of the original in a condensed form.

Writing a summary

- trains you to recognize the main points of an argument; and
- allows you to condense complex ideas into simple, clear points.

Some Special Types of Summaries

An **abstract** (see Box 2.3, p. 30) is a short overview of the main points of a document. Its purpose is to provide sufficient information for the reader to determine whether the article or book will be useful to his or her research. It is usually between 75 and 120 words in length and appears at the beginning of a document. When you are asked to write a research paper, you may be required to provide an abstract. For more information on writing an abstract, see page 48.

An **annotated bibliography** (see Box 2.4, p. 30) differs from a standard bibliography (list of references) in that it provides a brief description for each source listed. Its purpose is similar to that of an abstract.

Tips for Writing a Summary

1. Read the document once, from beginning to end. Do not summarize as you read; digest the entire piece of writing before attempting to summarize it.

BOX 2.1

Sample Article
Brain Rewiring: Using magnetic fields to treat depression is gaining favour

By Alexandra Shimo

Lying back in a spacious, leather armchair, Barbara Kwasniewski seems relaxed, especially given the nature of the medical treatment she's just received. The 53-year-old has undergone repetitive transcranial magnetic stimulation (rTMS), which essentially rearranges the pathways of the brain by using magnets.

The therapy was approved by Health Canada in 1997 and by the U.S. Food and Drug Administration in 2008. It's used to treat everything from strokes to depression, anorexia, migraines, obsessive-compulsive disorder, chronic pain and Parkinson's. It's one of a handful of therapies gaining popularity that use electricity to help rewire the brain. Deep brain stimulation is another, where wires are surgically implanted into a patient's grey matter to excite the neurons with electronic pulses. Electro-shock therapy has also made a comeback.

Of these electrical brain therapies, rTMS is the least invasive. Research is under way to determine its full potential: doctors aren't sure whether it's better to target one or both sides of the brain. They now stimulate just one side—the region depends on the disease—but this may change with further research. Nor have they determined how intense to make the magnetic field. If it's too strong, there is risk of causing a seizure. But if it's too weak, the treatment won't work. For these reasons, the therapy is regarded as experimental, says Dr. Gary Hasey, who started the first therapeutic transcranial magnetic stimulation lab in Canada in 1997.

What's groundbreaking about the treatment is that it can help people for whom all other options have failed. Studies show that about 40 per cent of these people improve, says Dr. Jeff Daskalakis, a psychiatrist who runs the brain treatment and research program at the University of Toronto. Kwasniewski fell into a deep depression 13 years ago, after giving birth to her daughter. She slept 18 or 20 hours per day. She tried every "antidepressant under the sun." Suicide was never far from her mind, and she would probably have gone through with it, she says, but for her daughter.

For the past three years, Kwasniewski has come to the Toronto-based Centre for Addiction and Mental Health (CAMH) for 20-minute sessions of rTMS. Twice a week, she sits in the big armchair. Next to the chair is a box with dials and knobs. Connected to the box is a black wire coil shaped like a figure eight. A nurse holds the coil to the top of Kwasniewski's head, just above the dorsolateral prefrontal cortex—an area of the brain responsible for planning and organization. When a current goes through the wire, it sets up a magnetic field, which is strongest at the point where the wires cross. The magnetic field excites the neurons underneath the coil, activating the pathways of her brain that inhibit negative thinking. The wire makes a clicking noise that sounds and feels, she says, like a woodpecker tapping at her skull. The known side effects of the treatment are seizures, headaches, and involuntary clenching of facial muscles, but so far, she's only suffered slight head pain after an early treatment.

In the public system, rTMS is available in Toronto, Hamilton, Vancouver, and Red Deer, but growing demand means the queues can be long; for example, at Toronto's CAMH, the wait is one year. The MindCare Centres offer the country's only private rTMS program, with clinics in Vancouver, Toronto, and Ottawa. A Montreal clinic opened just last week, and there's one more slated for Toronto. The cost is $5,000 to $7,500 for a course of treatment that lasts two to three weeks. The fees can be covered under insurance, although it's decided on a case-by-case basis. MindCare uses particularly strong magnets, setting the frequency above what has been tried in the research studies, and they report a higher success rate, with about 60 per cent of patients improving.

Every four months Bill Neill, 53, who lives in Oakbank, a suburb of Winnipeg, flies to Vancouver for a week of rTMS treatment at a MindCare Centre, which costs about $8,400 per year, including flights and hotels. Neill's doctors suggested he try rTMS because none of the anti-depressants eliminated his seasonal depression that was so serious that he used to take a leave from his job with Manitoba Hydro for a few months every year, and spend his days curled up in a ball, crying. He will probably need magnet therapy for the rest of his life, he says. "The cost is a stretch," says the father of three. "But it means I no longer live my life on a roller coaster." For Kwasniewski, the therapy has boosted her confidence and given her a renewed sense of purpose: her weight has fallen by 100 lb., and she has started to socialize again. Although there aren't any studies on how the therapy will affect her long-term health, she doesn't care. "If my brain turns to jelly in 20 years," she says partly in jest, "at least I will have had all those good years."

Source: " Brain rewiring," by Alexandra Shimo. Maclean's, *February 16, 2009.*

2. Read the document again, underlining or highlighting the main points, or noting the main points on a separate page.

3. Divide the document into sections; each section should have a main idea.

4. Write one sentence that captures the piece's main argument or thesis. This is your thesis statement; it should include the author's name, the title of the article, the topic of the original article, and the author's position on that topic.

5. Going through the article, compose one sentence for each section or main point and write them on a separate piece of paper.

6. Write one sentence that summarizes what can be learned from reading the article. This is your conclusion.

7. Read through your summary, checking for clarity, readability, and grammatical correctness. Check that you are not using the same wording as the author of the original text.

Note: For information on the distinction between summarizing and plagiarism, see pp. 62–63.

TRY IT YOURSELF

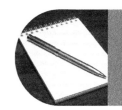

1. Read the article "Improve aboriginal health through oral history" (Box 2.5, p.31) and write a 100- to 200-word summary. Now, condense it even further into a 75–120 word abstract. Finally, write a 25–50 word annotated bibliography entry.

2. Choose a chapter or article in one of your textbooks and write a 100- to 200-word summary.

BOX 2.2 | A Summary of "Brain Rewiring"

In the article "Brain Rewiring" which appears on *Macleans.ca* on February 9, 2009, the author Alexandra Shimo discusses the use of transcranial magnetic stimulation (rTMS) to treat a number of medical conditions and describes how the therapy, so far, appears to be effective in treating depression. Shimo talks both to doctors who use the therapy and to patients who have reported success with using rTMS to treat their depression and raises some unanswered questions surrounding the therapy.

Repetitive transcranial magnetic stimulation, also known as rTMS, works by altering the brain's pathways through magnets. The treatment has been approved in both Canada and the U.S. and can be used to treat a variety of conditions including strokes, depression, obsessive compulsive disorder, chronic pain, and Parkinson's disease. While there are other electrical therapies available, rTMS is far less invasive than deep brain stimulation or electroconvulsive therapy. RTMS works by triggering the brain's neurons through the use of a magnetic field. This field, consequently, activates the part of the brain responsible for negative thinking.

While studies of the therapy's success, so far, indicate room for optimism, there are still some unanswered questions. Doctors are still unsure, for example, whether to apply the magnets on one or both sides of the brain and struggle with exactly how intense the magnetic field should be in order to be effective. In addition, the potential side effects of rTMS are seizures, headaches, and clenching of facial muscles. While the treatment is currently available in several Canadian cities, the waiting lists are long and the costs can be as high as $7 500. Still, for those who have undergone other treatment options for depression with little or no improvement, the author suggests that rTMS is a valid option.

BOX 2.3	An Abstract of "Brain Rewiring"

In the article "Brain Rewiring," Alexandra Shimo explains how repetitive transcranial magnetic stimulation, also known as rTMS, can be used to treat depression by altering the brain's pathways through magnets. The treatment has been approved in both Canada and the U.S. and can be used to treat a variety of conditions including strokes, depression, obsessive compulsive disorder, chronic pain, and Parkinson's disease. RTMS works by triggering the brain's neurons through the use of a magnetic field, which activates the part of the brain responsible for negative thinking. Shimo talks both to doctors who use the therapy and to patients who have reported success with using rTMS to treat their depression and raises some of the unanswered questions regarding the therapy.

BOX 2.4	An Annotated Bibliography Entry for "Brain Rewiring"

Shimo, A. (9 February, 2009). Brain rewiring. *Macleans.ca*. Retrieved June 12, 2009, from

   http://www2.macleans.ca/2009/02/09/brain-rewiring/

The author explains how repetitive transcranial magnetic stimulation, also known as rTMS, works by altering the brain's pathways through magnets. She describes how the treatment, so far, appears to be effective at treating depression, and discusses some of the drawbacks, such as long waiting times, high costs, and possible side effects.

THE CRITICAL ANALYSIS

A critical analysis (see Box 2.6) is, like a summary, a condensed version of a longer piece of writing. However, unlike a summary, an analysis includes your evaluation of what you have read. The goals in writing an analysis are (1) to give an objective explanation of a written text, and (2) to give your opinion on the author's views and on how successfully he or she has presented those views.

Writing a critical analysis

- trains you to read closely, and to understand what you read, rather than merely "skimming" the surface of a text;
- allows you to recognize the way a piece of writing is structured and to trace the development of the author's reasoning; and
- enables you to evaluate the strengths and weaknesses of an argument.

BOX 2.5

Sample Article
Improve aboriginal health through oral history

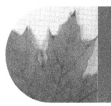

By Nicholas Keung

In 1965, a teenaged Rene Meshake was plucked away from his Aroland reserve in Northern Ontario and placed in a residential school.

For years, the Ojibway man suppressed his childhood memories of love, care, and indulgence because of the abuse and abandonment he experienced at the McIntosh and Fort Frances Indian schools.

"I remember the first rabbit I snared and skinned. Everybody just feasted on it. I was raised by the whole community," Meshake, now 62, recalls of his early years.

"But after the residential school, I was angry and depressed. I tried to block out all my memories by drinking," he said, pausing a moment. "I was afraid to trust again." Meshake later spent years being homeless in Toronto and often contemplated suicide.

Kim Anderson, a research associate with St. Michael's Hospital's Centre for Research on Inner City Health, said the residential school era not only disrupted the community's ability to build healthy relationships; it also robbed a generation of the opportunity to learn traditional parenting skills to raise their own healthy families, and ultimately contributed to the social ills faced by the community today.

"The residential school is the biggest and ugliest elephant in the middle of the room in terms of the disruptions," said the oral historian.

"Parenting skills were not passed on because there was no role modeling in these schools. We learn parenting by being parented. To top it all off, there was sexual and physical abuse. It added another dimension."

That is why Anderson has teamed up with colleague and family physician Dr. Janet Smylie—both are Métis—to establish the Indigenous Knowledge Network for Infant, Child and Family Health to uncover the lost traditions and develop culturally relevant health promotion strategies through aboriginal oral history.

"So far, European knowledge hasn't been making a big difference for aboriginal people. If you look at Northwestern Ontario, 30-plus of the communities over the last 15 years have seen a 20-fold expansion over access to western biomedicines—but their health outcomes are actually getting worse," said Smylie.

"Nobody is going to get better from a knowledge system that is very different from their own unless there is some kind of bridging. You have to work with people in a language and conceptual framework that fits for them," said Smylie. "Like any style of advertising and negotiation, you have to meet people where they are."

The five-year project involves 10 community partners in Ontario and Saskatchewan, where frontline health workers collect information from elders about lost skills and rituals in traditional parenting, pregnancy, labour and birth, and prenatal and postnatal care. They will then incorporate the knowledge in community health programming and practices.

Meshake was brought up by his grandparents and uncles, who taught him how to fish, hunt and live. All was good up until he was removed from the "res" (reserve).

He recalled his grandmothers would only wave a willow stick in front of his nose if he misbehaved, or use the threat of "Missabi" or Big Foot if he told a lie to teach him a lesson in honesty—a contrast to the stick beatings and strict discipline at the residential school.

When he left the residential school, Meshake never had a steady job or stable relationship and was rarely sober until he had an awakening in 1991.

"A friend of mine died. I went and buried him. I put the sand on his coffin and said to him, I'm burying my past with you," said Meshake, who has a graphic design diploma from Sheridan College and is now a published author and graphic artist.

"The residential school has disrupted the whole patterns of the rite of passage. This has to do with healing, sealing things," he said. "And I've told myself I would never pass on my negative experience to my (now 15-year-old) son."

Pauline Shirt, a Cree great-grandmother in Toronto, is more fortunate growing up at the Saddle Lake Reserve in Alberta. She too attended a residential school but remained close to her parents and nine siblings.

"I was raised on my father's farm to take care of Mother Earth and the animals. I learned about all the teachings of the spiritual world," said Shirt, 66, who helps raise her three great-grandchildren in Toronto.

"We believe in the seven stages of life where we each have our roles to play in the community. But unfortunately, a lot of people became disconnected and were robbed of those teachings."

As an elder, Shirt teaches traditional knowledge to others in the community. She also founded the First Nations School of Toronto in 1977, which was then called Wandering Spirit Survival School.

"We have to start with our youth," said Shirt. "We will need to help each other to help ourselves."

The project is funded by the Canadian Institutes of Health Research and Ontario Federation of Indian Friendship Centres.

Source: Nicholas Keung, "Improve aboriginal health through oral history." Toronto Star, May 2, 2010. reprinted with permission - Torstar Syndication Services.

Tips for Writing a Critical Analysis

1. Read the text.

2. Read it again, noting the following:

   - the author's purpose in writing (to inform, to persuade, to compare, etc.);
   - the intended audience; and
   - the topic, and the author's position on the topic.

3. Jot down the secondary arguments that support the main argument, along with the evidence used to support the arguments.

4. Ask yourself the following questions:

   - is the main argument of the piece clearly stated?;
   - is the organization of the piece logical?;
   - are the points well-supported?; and
   - has the author achieved his or her purpose?.

5. Write down the weaknesses of the author's argument. What points do you agree with? What points do you disagree with? Give reasons for both.

Structure of a Critical Analysis

Introduction

Your introduction should include the author's name, the title of the article or book, and the year in which it was published. It should also include the author's purpose, audience, and main argument. Last, it should also contain your thesis, which consists of your opinion about what you have read.

Summary

The next paragraph summarizes the main points that the author uses to support his or her argument. Provide an objective overview of the argument and supporting points. Do not give your opinion at this point.

Analysis

Now, evaluate the piece of writing. Is it convincing? Is there enough support? Is the support strong enough? How effective is it? Back up your opinions with evidence from the text itself.

Conclusion

End by briefly stating your overall evaluation of the piece. Is it effective, and why or why not? Has the author achieved his or her purpose? Is this article useful to the audience for which it is intended?

BOX 2.6

A Critical Analysis of "Brain Rewiring"

The article "Brain Rewiring" which appears on *Macleans.ca* on February 9, 2009, is written to inform the general public about a controversial new treatment for depression. Author Alexandra Shimo explains the use of repetitive transcranial magnetic stimulation (rTMS) to treat depression and other conditions. While Shimo provides moving testimonials from two patients currently undergoing rTMS treatment for severe depression, and consults two doctors who perform the treatment, this article does not adequately explore the science behind the therapy, the controversies surrounding the therapy, or the possible short- and long-term effects of the therapy.

As explained by Shimo, repetitive transcranial magnetic stimulation, also known as rTMS, works by altering the brain's pathways through magnets. The treatment has been approved in both Canada and the U.S. and can be used to treat a variety of conditions including strokes, depression, obsessive compulsive disorder, chronic pain, and Parkinson's disease. While there are other electrical therapies available, rTMS is far less invasive than deep brain stimulation or electroconvulsive therapy. RTMS works by triggering the brain's neurons through the use of a magnetic field. This field, consequently, activates the part of the brain responsible for negative thinking.

While studies of the therapy's success, so far, indicate room for optimism, there are still some unanswered questions. Doctors are still unsure, for example, whether to apply the magnets on one or both sides of the brain and struggle with exactly how intense the magnetic field should be in order to be effective. In addition, the potential side effects of rTMS are seizures, headaches, and clenching of facial muscles. While the treatment is currently available in several Canadian cities, the waiting lists are long and the costs can be as high as $7500. Still, for those who have undergone other treatment options for depression with little or no improvement, the author clearly feels that rTMS is a valid option.

In this article, Shimo focuses on the benefits of rTMS for treating depression; her evidence, however, is largely anecdotal, based on the experiences of two patients currently being treated with rTMS. Shimo's descriptions of how the treatment works are directed toward the non-specialist; the machine is described as "a box with dials and knobs," and the movement of the wire sounds and feels "like a woodpecker tapping at [the patient's] skull." Shimo mentions that there are questions regarding the intensity of the magnetic field, the best areas of the brain to target, and the short- and long-term side effects, but these are not pursued in her article. This article provides an overview of rTMS for a general readership and would be of very little use to health practitioners, other than as an introduction to the concept of rTMS.

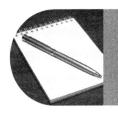

1. Read the article "Improve aboriginal health through oral history" and write a 200- to 400-word critical analysis.
2. Choose a chapter or article in one of your textbooks and write a 200- to 400-word critical analysis.

CONDUCTING RESEARCH

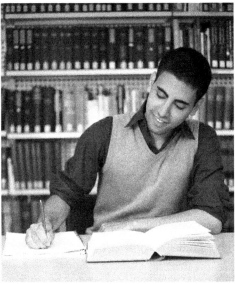

Robert Kneschke / Shutterstock

Locating information about a topic is an essential skill for both post-secondary education and your future career. While many students assume that the task of conducting research has been made easier by the proliferation of online encyclopedias, websites, and other online sources, it has actually been made more difficult. With an endless supply of information available, sorting out the useful, relevant, reliable sources of information from the rest can be an overwhelming task.

Where Should You Look?

Your **college or university library website** contains a wealth of resources. In addition to a catalogue of in-library resources, most library websites now provide access to the following:

- materials related to your specific course
- links to recommended websites
- databases of articles, listed by subject area
- style guides

- research help, including a live chat service
- online books, including dictionaries and encyclopedias

Do not simply enter your topic into Google or a similar search engine. Be sure to limit the choice to scholarly articles. **Google Scholar** (scholar.google.com, or select scholar from the main Google page) allows you to search peer-reviewed articles, dissertations, and books from cross-disciplinary academic sources. Similarly, **Academic Info** (academicinfo.net) is an online education resource centre which features a directory of links and resources arranged by subject area. According to the main page, the resources are compiled "taking into account their accessibility, authoritative sources as well as their ease of use, and aim to present a fair and well rounded perspective of the respective subject matter."

Why Does My Instructor Discourage the Use of Wikipedia?

A **wiki** is a website that anyone can contribute to or change. A site like Wikipedia is made up of millions of user-created, user-edited entries on an enormous range of topics. While the diversity of contributors does lead to a wide array of articles, and while the ability to edit others' contributions does mean that many inaccuracies are corrected, there is no formal mechanism for quality control. Also, the articles are general, as in an encyclopedia, and as such are not a source for specialized research or critical scholarship.

Many students rely on Wikipedia for their research, assuming that it is as reliable a source as traditional encyclopedias or reference books. It is true that Wikipedia can be a useful starting point for your research; however, in academic research, "peer-reviewed" sources are always preferable.

Peer review is a term for a selection process whereby articles are screened by experts in the field (professional "peers" of the article's author). If you were to submit an article about juvenile diabetes to a peer-reviewed journal or encyclopedia, your entry would be read by one or more people with a proven research record on similar subjects. If they found your research to be academically credible, the article would be published and future researchers would be able to consult it. If your article contained inaccuracies or faulty reasoning, or was otherwise poorly written, it would not be published.

Evaluating Online Sources

Ask yourself these questions to determine whether an online source is trustworthy:

1. What are the **author's qualifications and affiliations**? What makes him or her an authority on the subject? Is he or she biased? For example, an article on treatments for insomnia, written by the inventor of a new type of pillow for insomniacs, is not an objective source.

2. What is the **sponsoring organization** for the site? Is it a reputable organization? Is there a bias evident in the material? Is the site peer-reviewed? The site's domain

is often a clue to its affiliation: *.edu* indicates an educational institution, *.gov* indicates a government organization, and *.org* usually indicates a non-profit or non-commercial organization.

3. What is the **author's purpose** in writing? To inform? To persuade? To promote a product?

4. Does the site contain **current information**? How recently was the site updated? Are the links functional?

5. Are the sources on the site **properly documented**? Is there a list of works cited or references?

The Research Process, Step by Step

Your instructor has assigned you a research paper. The topic: Compare and contrast two similar chronic health conditions, their symptoms, and treatment options.

Step One:

This is a very broad topic, so the first step is to narrow it down. What type of conditions would you like to learn more about? Perhaps you are interested in asthma, which is a chronic lung condition. Because you are asked to both compare and contrast, you need to find another chronic lung condition that has both similarities to (compare) and differences from (contrast) asthma.

Wikipedia has no entries for "chronic lung conditions"; however, at the bottom of the Wikipedia entry on asthma is a section on "Differential Diagnosis" which mentions two conditions—chronic obstructive pulmonary disease and pulmonary aspiration—which closely resemble asthma. This gives you somewhere to begin.

Step Two:

Once you have narrowed down the topic enough to research further, it is time to search some reputable academic search engines, and to look at some of the resources available through your institution's library.

A search for "asthma or COPD" on Academic Info leads to the database MEDLINEplus, which informs readers of its objectivity: "There is no advertising on this site, nor does it endorse any company or product." The first five results include an article on the coexistence of asthma and COPD, published by the American Academy of Allergy, Asthma, and Immunology, and articles on the diagnosis and treatment of COPD and asthma, published by the National Lung Health Education Program. A search on Google Scholar brings up an article from the peer-reviewed journal *Chest*, by Peter J. Barnes, of the Department of Thoracic Medicine, National Heart and Lung Institute, London, UK, entitled "Mechanisms in COPD—Differences From Asthma." A couple of clicks confirm that *Chest* is the official journal of the American College of Chest Physicians and is the leading cardiopulmonary and critical care journal in the world. Add "Canada" to the search string and more articles, including many from

Chest, appear, including "Asthma Education: The Canadian Experience." The library home page of a typical college library provides links to a number of useful databases, including Academic Search Premier, ProQuest Nursing & Allied Health Source, Health Source: Nursing/Academic Edition, CINAHL (Cumulative Index to Nursing and Health Literature) and MEDLINEplus. Searches for "asthma and treatment or symptoms," and "chronic obstructive pulmonary disease or COPD and treatment or symptoms" result in many useful articles from books and refereed journals.

Step Three:

Now that you have located your sources, it is time to read them, looking for information that will support the claims that you are making in your essay or report. Keep a notebook or electronic file for keeping track of relevant quotations and examples to use. Be sure to write down the information about each source, including the page number, in order to make it easy for you to document your sources.

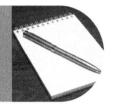

TRY IT YOURSELF

1. Choose one of the following terms and research it on (a) Google, (b) Wikipedia, (c) Google Scholar, and (d) on a database subscribed to by your college or university. Compare the results and evaluate their appropriateness as resources for a research essay or report.

Asperger syndrome	peptic ulcers	midwife
ADHD	echinacea	plantar wart

ESSAYS AND REPORTS

On your way to achieving the goal of being a skilled health professional, you first have to get through school. No matter what health science program you are enrolled in, it is highly unlikely that you will get through your program without having to write **essays** or **reports**.

What is the Difference between an Essay and a Report?

This is a very good question and one which is often debated among those who teach composition courses. While the answer to this question is open to interpretation, some differences are generally agreed upon. (See Table 2.1 on p. 39.)

Generally speaking, reports deal with facts and are experiment-oriented while essays are opinion-oriented. This means that courses that focus on critical thinking, like literature and philosophy, often expect essays while fact-based disciplines, like the sciences, encourage the writing of reports. Additionally, reports use **headings** to separate sections moreso than essays which tend to emphasize textual flow over section breaks. Table 2.1 contrasts common section requirements of essays and reports.

TABLE 2.1   Contrasting the Essay and the Academic Report

	THE ESSAY	THE FORMAL ACADEMIC REPORT
PRESENTATION OF GOAL	Thesis statement	Purpose statement Objective
PARTS	Title page Introduction Body Conclusion References (if research essay)	Title page Abstract Table of Contents List of Figures List of Tables Introduction Literature Review Methods and Materials Results Discussion References Tables Figure Captions Figures Appendices Note: The exact sections required will be determined by the professor
SECTION BREAKS	Topic sentences	Headings
MISCELLANEOUS	Emphasized in the humanities	Emphasized in the sciences

A common type of report found in the health sciences is a classification report. A classification report might ask you to classify fast food items in terms of fat content. In a report on this topic, your goal is to present facts, in a structured and organized way, and then interpret these facts analytically and meaningfully.

Sometimes, however, your professors will require that you write an essay instead of a report. A persuasive essay, for example, is a commonly asked for academic essay (see Box 2.7 on p. 40). A student might, for example, be asked to argue his or her

BOX 2.7 **Sample Persuasive Essay**

Demanding Transparency from the Fast Food Industry

Notice how the introductory paragraph moves from general to specific and how the thesis appears as the last sentence. The thesis sets up the writer's argument clearly and assertively and provides the order of details that follow.

A transition is used to segue into the opening body paragraph.

The topic sentence introduces the main point of the first body paragraph: convenience.

The use of transition here, is consistent with usage in the paragraph above.

The topic sentence introduces the main point of the second body paragraph: education.

A rhetorical question can be an effective way to engage the reader with your topic.

It is always important to answer your critics, particularly in a persuasive essay where you are trying to convince others of your opinion.

Current food trends in Canada clearly point to a country where health and well-being matter. From the growing organics food industry to packed exercise clubs, outdoor boot camps, and the numerous diet books sold in bookstores, looking good and feeling healthy seem to be a priority for many Canadians. To further this trend, there has been recent discussion in Canada concerning the implementation of laws that would require fast food restaurants to post nutritional information about the foods they sell. Canada should, indeed, enact nation-wide laws that require fast food restaurants to post nutritional information about their food products for three very good reasons: convenience, education, and health.

First, having access to nutritional information at the point of purchase is a convenient and effective way of providing consumers with important health information. In a 24/7 society, where banking and grocery shopping can be done at virtually any time, it seems that Canadians demand convenience, especially in urban areas where time is of the essence. The busy professional often finds him- or herself in a situation of having to "pick up" a snack or a meal, and the convenience of fast food restaurants, coupled with their affordability, makes fast food a practical option for many. While consumers might be able to access nutritional information about their favourite fast foods online, when craving a McDonald's Big Mac or a Dairy Queen Blizzard, it is very doubtful that an individual will first "log in" in order to determine the fat content or caloric information of their favourite treat. The immediacy of nutritional information that is visible and accessible at the point of purchase may very well be the factor that motivates a consumer to make a healthier food choice.

Second, in a democratic society it is only right that citizens be educated on the foods that they ingest. While ignorance can be bliss, when it starts to affect health, knowledge is preferable. Canadians demand transparency in many aspects of their lives, including what politicians spend taxpayer dollars on as well as what kids are being taught in school, so it is only right that we expect restaurants to be transparent about the content of the foods they serve. If nutritional information reveals that a typical serving of soda contains 40 grams of sugar, would you still choose to ingest it? The fact is that while a good number of Canadians want to eat healthier, words like "monounsaturated" and "unsaturated" and the percent-ages and calculations that often appear on nutritional information tables seem to be a secret code that only a select few can interpret. Educating consumers on how to interpret nutrition labels as well as informing consumers, in an accessible way, about the nutritional content of popular fast food products like burgers, fries, and milkshakes might inspire healthier food choices. Some critics bring up the notion of free will and suggest that restaurants should not be forced to post such information. Despite the democratic principles that flourish in Canada, businesses are required to abide by laws all the time, sanitation and zoning laws, for example, so the argument against coercion is not a realistic one. The free will of the consumer would certainly not be affected by mandatory posting of nutritional information as it is the consumer who ultimately chooses, despite the posting of the information, whether to consume a product or not. In fact, the consumer is the one who makes the choice as to whether he or she even wishes to read the nutritional information in the first place.

Third, obesity appears to be a growing problem in North America and making it mandatory for fast food restaurants to post nutritional information may help in efforts to reduce obesity and other health complications associated with it. Obesity has been linked to poor self-esteem and bullying (particularly in youngsters) as well as serious health complications like heart disease and hypertension. Consumers concerned about obesity or health risks associated with the regular consumption of fast foods may, indeed, select healthier items if provided with information on a particular's food's nutritional value, or lack thereof. By accessing such information, consumers are able to make more informed choices. A comprehensive listing of a food's ingredients can also save individuals with food sensitivities great distress or possibly even death. Critics may argue that it has not been proven that the posting of such information would decrease obesity rates. However, it also has not been proven that such information would not curb obesity rates. As such, if the transparency of fast food nutritional content has the potential to make Canadians healthier, it seems reasonable to, at least, give it a try.

In conclusion, some states in the U.S. have already started to experiment with the mandatory posting of nutritional information at fast food restaurants and Canada should as well. Convenient access to health information as well as transparency in what we ingest has the potential to lead to healthier food choices, and healthier food choices may help in efforts to curb obesity and those ailments associated with it. While a law proposing the mandatory listing of nutritional information at fast food establishments is not an all-encompassing and easy fix to problems concerning health and well-being, and would require significant planning, administration, and confrontations with "nay-sayers", the government should still take the time and effort to implement such measures based on the potential benefits that may arise. Given all the potential advantages of posting nutritional information, it is difficult to understand why nation-wide laws supporting it have not already been implemented.

A third opening transition is used here.

The topic sentence introduces the main point of the third body paragraph: health.

The author, again, answers her critics here, providing further strength and validity to her argument in the process.

The transition "In conclusion" signals that the essay is about to come to a close.

The summary statement restates the author's thesis and appears at the beginning of the concluding paragraph.

The author closes with a thought-provoking statement.

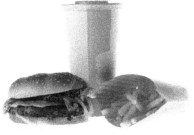

Mariola Kraczowska/ Shutterstock

perspective on a debatable topic, like the mandatory listing of nutritional information on all fast food menus.

Unlike the classification report mentioned earlier, where your goal is to provide factual information, here your purpose is to take a stance on whether nutritional information should be listed, or not, on fast food menus. If your essay requires research, you would also have to integrate credible sources that support your particular stance on the subject.

THE ACADEMIC ESSAY: INTRODUCTION, BODY, AND CONCLUSION

The Introduction

The first paragraph in an essay is called the **introductory paragraph**. This paragraph introduces your topic as well as your viewpoint on the topic. Introductory paragraphs should go from general to specific: they begin by providing some general background on the topic, often through the form of definitions and other information that helps establish context. The essay introduction is the first thing your reader sees so make sure it effectively and accurately represents the contents of your essay. The most important part of the essay introduction, however, is the **thesis statement**.

DON'T

- include specific examples or details in your introduction.
- stray from the essay topic.

The Thesis Statement

The thesis statement expresses your argument or your opinion on the topic that you are writing about. In undergraduate courses, professors usually encourage students to place their thesis statement at the end of the introductory paragraph. This means that the thesis statement is the most specific part of your introduction, recalling from our earlier discussion that the introduction flows from general to specific. While many students fear the thesis statement, writing one does not have to be intimidating or scary if you remember this simple, no-fail formula:

$$Essay\ topic + viewpoint = thesis$$

Suppose, for example, that your professor wants you to write an essay based on the following essay topic:

Discuss the special predicaments male nurses face in the hospital setting.

The first step in creating a thesis based on this topic is to plug the right variables into the no-fail formula:

Topic = special predicaments of male nurses

Your viewpoint = male nurses are stereotyped, discriminated against and have a lack of support

Then, combine the two parts together:

Male nurses in hospitals have to battle the following challenges: stereotypes, discrimination, and lack of psychological support.

You have just created a thesis statement.

If you look carefully at the above statement, you will notice that you not only created a thesis in response to the topic, but you did another very important thing in the process: you set up the organization of your paper. Your thesis statement shows that your first body paragraph will deal with how male nurses are stereotyped, your second body paragraph will deal with how male nurses are discriminated against, and your third body paragraph will deal with how male nurses lack support to deal with their specific challenges.

So, good thesis statements do at least two things: they express your argument clearly and concisely, and set up the organization of the piece of writing that follows.

Now that you understand what a good thesis statement is, it is equally important to avoid creating a bad one by paying close attention to the "Don't" list below.

DON'T

- write an announcement

  In this essay, I will...

  The subject of this essay is...

- write a thesis that is too broad for the length restrictions of your assignment

  All the paramedic programs at colleges around the world have high standards.

- state a fact

  Canada's health care system is publicly funded.

- argue points that are not unique and distinct

  Wrong: *Regular cardio exercise benefits an individual's physical health, bone health, and emotional health.*

  In the statement above, the thesis points are not unique and distinct as bone health is part of overall physical heath. So, you need to rewrite your statement making sure your thesis items are unique and distinct.

Right: *Regular cardio exercise benefits an individual's physical health and emotional health.*

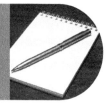

TRY IT YOURSELF

1. Indicate whether the following statements are good thesis statements for a 1000-word essay. Be prepared to defend your choice.

   a) There are problems with Canada's health care system.
   b) I will write about how H1N1 flu is spread.
   c) Common triggers for anorexia nervosa include low self-esteem, media influence, and dysfunctional relationships.
   d) Male nurses encounter more workplace challenges than female nurses.
   e) To be a successful paramedic one must be flexible, adaptable, and able to handle change.

The Body

All paragraphs within your essay with the exception of the opening and closing paragraphs constitute the essay **body**. The body of an essay is where you showcase the evidence and examples that support your thesis. The length of your essay's body depends upon the specific requirements of your assignment, but undergraduate programs are fond of the five paragraph model for shorter essays, which means that there are three body paragraphs framed by both an introduction and a conclusion. Each body paragraph must have a **topic sentence**. A topic sentence is a statement which appears at the beginning of each new paragraph and explains the contents of that particular paragraph.

Organization of the Body

As you attempt to organize your thoughts and sort through what appears to be a mountain of information that you wish to express about your topic, you have to tackle the problem of how to best organize all this information. Four common methods of organizing body paragraphs are listed here.

- Work Chronologically

  This type of structure works well for essays in which time sequence or chronology matters. If you are writing about the evolution of breast cancer treatment, it would make sense to begin with older treatments and then work up to more modern day ones.

- Work Climactically

  Like the long distance runner who chooses to start a marathon slowly in order to conserve energy for a strong finish, authors often choose to end their essays with what they determine to be their strongest point in order to leave a memorable impression on the reader.

- Work Logically

  In certain topics, the logic of an essay is obvious. For example, if you are writing a process essay on how to insert a contact lens, it would be illogical to begin with the final step, where you put your contact solution back into the bathroom cabinet.

- Work Randomly

  Sometimes body organization is nothing more than authorial preference. If there is no apparent pattern to your points or no perceived advantage in organizing according to a theme or pattern, the random ordering of main points is acceptable.

DON'T

- include material in your essay's body that does not aid you in your argument or that does not support your thesis.
- repeat information in the different body paragraphs.

TRY IT YOURSELF

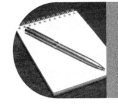

1. Suppose you are writing a five-paragraph essay based on each of the thesis statements below. What would your three topic sentences be for each thesis statement?

   a) The advantages of computerized record-keeping in hospitals include efficiency, accuracy, and service enhancement.
   b) The patient-client relationship is centred on trust, patience, and responsibility.
   c) Better education as to what constitutes an emergency, an increase in the number of emergency rooms, and presence of more trained hospital staff can help decrease waiting times in Toronto emergency rooms.
   d) The Bachelor of Nursing degree is intense, educational, and marketable.
   e) Elder abuse, improperly trained personnel, and overworked staff are three rampant problems in Canadian nursing homes.

Conclusion

The last paragraph of your essay is your conclusion. It is the last part of the essay that your reader sees, so it should leave a memorable impression. The first sentence of your conclusion is known as a **summary statement** and restates (not copies) your thesis. The summary statement signals closure for the reader.

DON'T

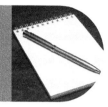

- introduce new ideas or new arguments in the conclusion.

TRY IT YOURSELF

Jody Moritsugu's essay "The Beauty of Blogs" (Box 2.8) in its original form is a five-paragraph essay. In the revision below, however, it has been written as one long paragraph. See if you can find the starting and end points for the various essay sections that have been discussed so far.

BOX 2.8 **The Beauty of Blogs**

By Jody Moritsugu

"Blog": such an ugly word to describe a beautiful and powerful phenomenon. A blog—short for "weblog"—is a personal, professional, or political journal that is posted on the Internet. The activity of maintaining a blog is known as "blogging"; "bloggers" are people who write online dissections of subjects ranging from Alberta and Alzheimer's to Zaire and Zambonis; and the "blogosphere" is the community of all blogs on the World Wide Web. What explains the growing international audience for blogs? The news blogs that I participate in provide some clues: they present a forum for stimulating, immediate, and democratic communication that is increasingly missing from conventional media. You might think that reading other people's opinions is boring, but if a blog is well researched and well written, the ideas it presents can be illuminating. A good blogger pays close attention to the news of the day—a time-consuming task in our information-saturated world—and then publishes an alternative analysis: interpreting, making connections, and drawing conclusions not found in mainstream sources. The blogs I read often contain information not covered by traditional news media, partly because of time and space limitations imposed on network news outlets and partly because of political restrictions. The Internet has no such limits or restrictions. One of the most appealing features of blogs is their immediacy. Blogs are dynamic, real-time sources of information. Bloggers can respond virtually instantly to any event; some routinely post their opinions several times a day. The liveliest blogs give readers the opportunity to post their own messages—messages that, unlike the letters to the editor found in traditional print media, are not edited for content or length. The opportunity for online dialogue engages readers more deeply than the one-way communication offered by mass media. Beyond the immediacy and ever-changing forum of ideas and information they offer, blogs have the potential to be vehicles for genuine democracy. Blogging is revolutionizing the way people worldwide get and distribute information. In stark contrast to the authoritarian, "voice of God" stance adopted by most mass media, blogs encourage a wide range of voices to speak up and be heard. Bloggers can post anything they wish (so long as they observe the laws governing hate messages or child pornography, for example). In the blogosphere, there are no gatekeepers to distort or limit information, no editors to chop your prose to pieces, no owners whose political biases must be catered to. Such unfettered freedom of speech is not without risk, but once you learn how to separate the well-informed, trustworthy blogs from the uninformed rubbish—and there is lots of it—you gain access to dynamic, thought-provoking media sources that can be just as (if not more) reliable than the increasingly scandal-plagued traditional print and electronic media. Good blogs are intellectually challenging, dynamic, and current. They provide forums for debate and discussion, a precondition for democracy. Blogs give ordinary people like you and me the power of information and the opportunity to share our opinions with the rest of the world.

Source: From Norton/Green, Essay Essentials with Readings, *Nelson Education Ltd., 2006. Reprinted by permission.*

The thesis statement is:

_____

The topic sentence of the first paragraph is:

_____

The topic sentence of the second paragraph is:

_____

The topic sentence of the third paragraph is:

_____

The topic sentence of the fourth paragraph is:

_____

The summary statement is:

_____

APA STYLE

In the next section, you will come across many references to "APA style." APA style refers to the standard academic paper format that is endorsed by the American Psychological Association (APA) and used in the sciences and social sciences. Since 1929, the APA has published a set of guidelines for preparing a scholarly paper; a paper prepared according to these guidelines meets the criteria for consideration for publication in a professional journal in the sciences or social sciences. The APA style conventions for the format of the essay or report will be covered on pp. 55–56. The APA guidelines for documenting sources are covered on pp. 57–61.

WRITING IN AN ACADEMIC SETTING

THE ACADEMIC REPORT

As mentioned previously, there is no "one size fits all" model for either the essay or the academic report: report organization and content is dependent on the requirements of a particular discipline, course, and instructor.

In preparing an academic report, you may be asked to conduct **primary research** whereby you conduct your own study or experiment, and then present your findings, or you may be asked to do **secondary research** where you analyze and interpret the research of others. Below you will find definitions and explanations for common report sections in APA style papers. Your instructor will tell you which sections he or she wants you to incorporate.

Abstract

The Abstract appears after the **title page** (see page 66) and is a brief summary of the major points of your report. As the Abstract summarizes your report, it allows a reader to quickly determine whether to read further, or not. The Abstract follows the title page and appears on a page by itself. It is a maximum of 120 words long and is written in block (not indented) format. Even though the Abstract is one of the first report sections the reader sees, it is often the last thing written.

Table of Contents

The Table of Contents is a listing of your report's contents and is particularly valuable for quickly finding information in long reports. It includes the section headings and page numbers of the various parts of your report. The Table of Contents follows the Abstract. Do not include the title page as an item in your Table of Contents.

List of Tables

The List of Tables is similar to the Table of Contents except that it lists the title and page numbers of any tables you have incorporated into your report. The List of Tables follows the Table of Contents in your report.

List of Figures

The List of Figures is similar to the Table of Contents except that it lists the title and page numbers of any figures you have incorporated into your report. The List of Figures follows the List of Tables in your report.

Introduction

This section outlines the purpose and scope of your study, experiment or analysis. The heading "Introduction" is not used in APA: material placed at the beginning of your report is understood to be introductory. Whether your report is based on a study or experiment or you are writing an informational piece, you must have a **purpose statement** or **objective**: a clear and focused goal which is articulated at the outset of the report. The purpose statement in a report serves the same function as a thesis in an essay: it tells the reader what the purpose or goal of the report is. Like the thesis statement, it should be clear, focused, and expressive of the report's contents.

Review of Literature

A literature review appears at the beginning of a report and summarizes and evaluates the significant literature that you have looked at in preparing your report. You do not have to include all the sources that you have read; rather, the sources you choose for comment should be organized around the central purpose of your paper. Ultimately, a good literature review shows that the author has done comprehensive background reading and research on his or her topic; as well, the review provides context for the information and research which is to come.

Materials and Method

If your report is based on primary research, you will need to include a Materials and Method section. Here, you describe the set-up of your study as well as the techniques you used to acquire the data contained in your report. Methods of experimentation and data collection are discipline-specific, so will vary, but commonly include things like questionnaires, interviews, and focus groups. Your description of the materials and methods used in your study must be detailed and comprehensive.

Results

This section details the presentation of your findings. It is important to note that the data you present here should be stated objectively and should not be commented on or analyzed. Tables and figures are a convenient and effective way to present study results and are often included in this section.

Discussion

In this section, you interpret and comment on the findings presented in the Results section. The Discussion is the place to comment on notable patterns or relationships that connect to your original purpose or objective. Additionally, you should connect your personal findings to any existing research. Any problems or gaps with your methods and/or materials should also be commented on and recommendations for further research should be made.

References

This section details the sources that you have paraphrased, summarized or quoted in your report and appears at the end of your document. Entries are double-spaced and listed alphabetically according to the last name of the author. Books, magazines, and websites are all cited differently (see page 68). The first line of each entry begins at the left-hand margin; second and subsequent lines are indented five to seven spaces.

Tables

Tables should be placed after the References section. Each table should be on its own page. Make sure your tables are labelled consecutively and you follow correct rules for formatting captions (see page 52).

Figure Captions

The Figure Captions page follows any tables and lists all the captions for the figures used in your report (see page 52).

Figures

Any figures you have used should be placed after the Figure Captions page. Each figure should be placed on a separate page.

Appendix

Some reports also include an Appendix. This section follows the References section. An Appendix contains material which is referred to in the text of the report but has been determined to be distracting or awkward if placed within the main text. Your Appendix should include only those items that enhance your report's message. Common items found in an Appendix include photos, drawings, charts, and graphs.

HEADINGS IN APA STYLE

Headings help with the organization of information as well as determine the hierarchy of information in your report. The number of heading levels used depends on the number of categories and sub-categories in your report. The 6th edition of the APA manual stresses the following five-level heading structure.

Level 1 – **Centred, Bold, Standard Capitalization**

Level 2 – **Flush left, Bold, Standard Capitalization**

Level 3 – **Indented, bold, lowercase, period at the end.**

Level 4 – ***Indented, bold, italicized, lowercase, period at the end.***

Level 5 – *Indented, italicized, lowercase, period at the end.*

Most papers at an undergraduate level will not require more than three different heading levels. In order to incorporate headings correctly, you must first determine how many different heading levels you will need. Once you have done this, follow the guidelines below:

- If you have one level of title, use Level 1 only.
- If you have two levels of titles, use Levels 1 and 2.
- If you have three levels of titles, use Levels 1, 2, and 3.
- If you have four levels of titles, use Levels 1, 2, 3, and 4.
- If you have five levels of titles, use Levels 1, 2, 3, 4, and 5.

USING VISUALS IN YOUR REPORT

Visuals in reports can be greatly beneficial. They concentrate information and allow for complex ideas to be expressed creatively and efficiently. In the APA style, visuals are divided into two categories: tables and figures. Tables are instantly recognizable by rows and columns that contain either numerical data or text (matrix). A figure, on the other hand, refers to any type of visual that is not a table. This includes graphs, charts, drawings, and photographs.

APA Standards for Both Figures and Tables

According to APA guidelines, when using visuals in academic reports, you should follow the standards below:

- Any visual used must be referred to in your text.
- Figures should complement, rather than duplicate, textual information.
- All figures and tables are numbered consecutively with Arabic numerals (e.g., Figure 1, Figure 2, Table 1, Table 2).
- You must cite the source for your visual in your References page. Such citations are similar to those used for books. See pp. 69–72.
- Manuscript style dictates that visuals should be placed at the end of the report (after the References page but before the Appendix). Each table and figure is placed on a separate page; a Figure Captions page, which lists the captions of all the figures used, precedes the figures section.
- Figure and table placement in undergraduate or non-published works depends on instructor preference. Your professor may require that a visual be placed on a separate page immediately following its first reference or that it be directly incorporated into the body of the essay or report.
- If you are using a non-original table or figure, include a note under your visual providing enough source information for it to be traced to your References page.

Figure Captioning: the Specifics

- The word "Figure" and its respective number should be italicized with a period after it. Capitalize only first words and proper nouns in figure captions. The caption is followed by a period.
- Unlike table captions, which are placed above a table, figure captions appear on a separate page as explained on pp. 71–72.

FIGURE 2.1 | **Sample Figure and Caption**

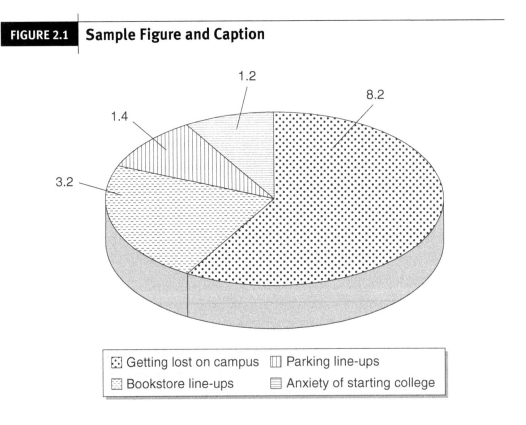

Figure 1. Top four frustrations as reported by a random sampling of Lester College students the first week of classes.

(*Ross, 2006, p. 12*)

Table Captioning: the Specifics

- The word "Table" along with its respective number appears on a line by itself. The table caption is italicized with significant words capitalized. The entire caption is placed above the visual. A double-space separates the table heading from the table caption. See example below.

TABLE 2.2	**Sample Table and Caption**

Table 6:   A Sample Food Diary Template From Sunflower Health Clinic

	BREAKFAST	LUNCH	DINNER	SNACK
SUNDAY				
MONDAY				
TUESDAY				
WEDNESDAY				
THURSDAY				
FRIDAY				
SATURDAY				

(Edgell, 2007, p. 57)

TRY IT YOURSELF

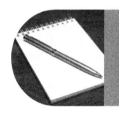

See how well you understand the APA standards for figure and table captioning. Write captions for each of the visuals in Figures 2.2, 2.3, 2.4, and Table 2.3, following all proper rules of spacing, formatting, and capitalization.

FIGURE 2.2	**Caption Exercise #2**

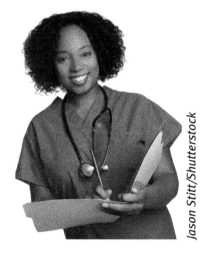

Jason Stitt/Shutterstock

Nursing:

A REWARDING

CAREER

FIGURE 2.3 **Caption Exercise #3**

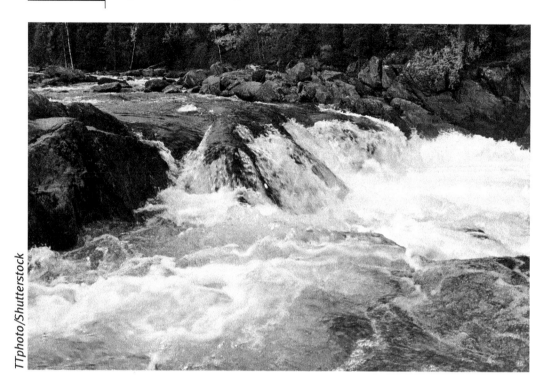

TTphoto/Shutterstock

FIGURE 2.3 **Caption Exercise #3**

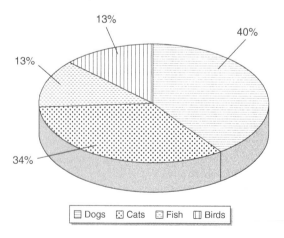

13%

40%

13%

34%

☐ Dogs ☒ Cats ☐ Fish ☐ Birds

TABLE 2.3	Caption Exercise #4

NUMBER	SQUARE	CUBE	SQUARE ROOT OF NUMBER
1	1	1	1.000
2	4	8	1.414
3	9	27	1.732
4	16	64	2.000
5	25	125	2.236
6	36	216	2.449
7	49	343	2.645
8	64	512	2.828
9	81	729	3.000
10	100	1000	3.162
11	121	1331	3.316
12	144	1728	3.464
13	169	2197	3.605
14	196	2744	3.741
15	225	3375	3.872
16	256	4096	4.000
17	289	4913	4.123
18	324	5832	4.242
19	361	6859	4.358
20	400	8000	4.472

APA FORMAT GUIDELINES FOR ESSAYS AND REPORTS

In addition to understanding the parts that make up an essay or a report, you must also follow correct APA formatting procedures. The following guidelines reflect basic APA formatting principles.

- Type your essay on 8½ by 11-inch white paper and use one side of the paper only.
- Double-space throughout your assignment.

- Leave 1-inch margins at the top, bottom, and sides of each page.
- Do not justify the right margin; leave it ragged.
- The APA does not like underlining. Use italics throughout.
- Type your essay in a 12-point typeface like Times Roman, Arial, or Courier.
- Staple your essay or report in the top left corner. Binders and folders are often discouraged, but check with your instructor.
- Use Arabic numbers when numbering pages.
- Formal essays and reports must have a **title page**. The title page includes the full report title, along with the author's name, course, professor, and date of submission (see sample report on page 65). Make sure your essay or report title clearly describes the contents of your report. Do not put visuals on your title page.
- All pages of your report, with the exception of the title page, must include a **page header,** a shortened version of the essay or report title, as well as a page number. The page header should be placed at the top of the page flush left, while page numbers are placed flush right.
- While the title page does not include a page header, it must include a **running head**. The running head lists either the full or abbreviated title of the essay or report and is typed in uppercase letters. Abbreviated titles should be used when the original title is longer than 50 characters. The running head is flush left and appears in the top corner of the title page.

THE WRITING PROCESS

While there is no set way of approaching the task of writing a research essay or report, it is important to have some system of organization, or you may feel overwhelmed by what is expected of you. Consider the following approach, in the suggested order, as you plan and organize your research essay or research report.

- Choose a topic from the choices offered to you.
- Research your topic. Stay clearly focused on the issue at hand, or you will end up having to sort through too much information. Record bibliographical data like authors, titles, and page numbers of any sources you feel are relevant to your purpose. This information is vital when it comes time to do your in-text citations and References page.
- Once you have done some preliminary research, establish your thesis or purpose statement. Based on the knowledge you have and the research and reading that you have undertaken, you should have a clearly defined argument or perspective.
- Sort through the information you have recorded from your research, and use any quotes, facts, opinions, or statistics that specifically support your thesis or purpose.
- Compose an outline. Keep in mind that you will most likely have to adapt this outline as you embark on the writing process.
- Write at least two rough drafts, remembering to integrate information you found during the research process, and correctly citing all "outside" ideas with in-text references. Then, prepare your final copy complete with a References page.

DOCUMENTING SOURCES IN APA STYLE

When you use sources to support your arguments, you need to document them properly. The two main documentation styles in North America are MLA (Modern Language Association) in the humanities, and APA (American Psychological Association) in the sciences and social sciences. Documentation in APA style consists of two components: in-text citations and a list of references.

Because the rules for APA documentation are very complex, we will cover the basic rules and most common student errors. For more detailed information, please consult one of the following:

- The APA Guide at the Online Writing Lab at Purdue University

    http://owl.english.purdue.edu/owl/section/2/10/

- APA Style

    http://www.apastyle.org/

- APA Style on Twitter

    http://twitter.com/APA_Style

- Dalhousie University's Quick Guide

    http://www.library.dal.ca/Files/How_do_I/pdf/apa_style6.pdf

- In addition, your college or university may have a reference tool such as RefWorks that allows you to create your list of references easily as you research. Visit your library or refer to its website for more information.

In-Text Citations

The term "in-text citation" refers to a reference that is contained in the body of your essay. When you quote or paraphrase material from an external source, you are required to let the reader know where you obtained the material. Box 2.9 addresses frequently asked questions on APA in-text citations.

Quotations

When you quote material directly from a source within your paper, you need to indicate the source. In APA format, this is done using the author-date-page method; the author's last name, the date of publication, and the page number (if available) must appear in the text, either in the sentence preceding the quotation or in parentheses after the quotation.

Example:

Roy Ashmeade fought the Ontario government for access to Vidaza, which "was the only treatment that held the hope of extending his life after he was diagnosed with myelodysplastic syndrome, which occurs when blood-forming cells in the bone marrow are damaged" (Priest, 2009, A8).

In his 2009 article, Priest documents Roy Ashmeade's fight with the Ontario government for access to Vidaza, which "was the only treatment that held the hope of extending his life after he was diagnosed with myelodysplastic syndrome, which occurs when blood-forming cells in the bone marrow are damaged" (A8).

Note: If there are quotation marks, they should precede the parentheses. Other punctuation (period, comma, etc.) should follow the parentheses.

BOX 2.9 **APA IN-TEXT CITATIONS F.A.Q.**

1. What do I do if there is no author listed for an article I'm using? What do I do if there's no date listed?

   - When a source has no named author, cite the first few words of the title. Italicize titles of books or reports; put titles of articles in quotation marks.

   ("Breathe Easy", 2003)

2. A lot of the sources I'm using have more than one author. Do I need to list all of them?

   - For a work with two authors, cite both names every time you refer to the work.

   - For a work with three to five authors, cite all the names the first time you refer to the work; for all other references to the work, cite only the first author, followed by *et al.* (the abbreviation of *et alia*, which is Latin for "and the others").

   - First reference: (Canning, Courage, & Frizzell, 2004)

   - All future references: (Canning, et al., 2004)

   - For a work with six or more authors, cite only the name of the first author, followed by *et al.*

3. I'm using two books written by the same author. How do I distinguish between them?

   - Include the year of publication in the citation. This will help your reader identify the source. If both sources are published in the same year, use the lower-case letters a, b, c, and so on, to distinguish between them.

   (Barnes, 2003) (Barnes, 2005a) (Barnes 2005b)

4. I'm using an online source and can't find page numbers. What do I do?

   - For sources that lack page numbers, use the abbreviation "para." or the symbol ¶ followed by the paragraph number. You could also provide a section heading, plus the paragraph number within the section. Do not use the page numbers of printed web pages.

   (Barnes, 2003, para. 25)

Paraphrases

A paraphrase is a restatement of the content of a text, using different words. When you are paraphrasing or summarizing material from a source, only the author's name and the date need to be provided.

Example:

Roy Ashmeade, diagnosed with myelodysplastic syndrome, fought the Ontario government for access to Vidaza, a drug that could possibly have prolonged his life (Priest, 2009).

List of References

The in-text citations are intended to direct readers to the more complete list of references at the end of the paper. All sources cited in the paper must appear in the list of references. (See Box 2.10 for answers to frequently asked questions.) Your References list should be double spaced, and should begin on a separate page, with the title "References" centred at the top of the page. See the sample References list in Box 2.11 (p. 61).

Consult the online sources listed on p. 57 for more detailed instructions.

BOX 2.10   **APA REFERENCE PAGE F.A.Q.**

1. What do I do if there is no author listed for an article I'm using? What do I do if there's no date listed?

   - If no author is given, begin the entry with the title of the source. List the source alphabetically by the first letter of the first word (not including "a" or "the") of the title.

   Breathe easy: Good nutrition can help keep your lungs healthy. (June 2003). *Environmental Nutrition* 26 (6). Retrieved April 22, 2009, from AltHealthWatch.

   - If no date is given, use the abbreviation "n.d." (for "no date") where the date would be.

   World Health Organization (n.d.) *International travel and health*. Retrieved June 18, 2009, from http://www.who.int/ith/en/index.html

2. A lot of the sources I'm using have more than one author. In what order do I list the authors? How do I separate the names?

   - List the authors in the same order that they are listed on the title page of the book or the first page of the article. Do not alphabetize the names. Use an ampersand (&)

---

instead of the word "and" when separating authors' names. For entries with more than two authors, separate the names by commas and place an ampersand before the last name of the last author listed.

Berlin, L., Albertsson, D.; Bengtsson Tops, A., Dahlberg, K., & Grahn, B. (July 2009). Elderly women's experiences of living with fall risk in a fragile body: A reflective lifeworld approach. *Health & Social Care in the Community, 17* (4), 379–387.

3. I'm confused about quotation marks, underlining, and italics. When do I use each one?

- Italicize titles of longer works (books, encyclopedias, journals, newspapers, movies, etc.)

- Do not italicize, underline, put quotation marks around, or distinguish in any other way the titles of shorter works (articles, essays, poems, stories, etc.)

Lewis, S. (2008). Pandemic: My country is on its knees. In Ackley, K.A., Blank, G.K. Hume, S.E. *Perspectives on contemporary issues: Reading across the disciplines* (274-390). Toronto: Nelson.

Bartlett, S., LeRose, M., & Ridout, S. (Producers), & Bartlett, S. & Le Rose, M. (Directors). (2008). *Desperately seeking doctors* [Motion picture].Canada: Dreamfilm Productions Inc. & the Canadian Broadcasting Corporation.

Canning, P.M., Courage, M.L., & Frizzell, L.M. (2004, August 3), Prevalence of overweight and obesity in a provincial population of Canadian preschool children. *CMAJ: Canadian Medical Association Journal*, Vol. 171 (3). Retrieved from Health Source: Nursing / Academic Edition.

4. What words do I capitalize?

- All major words in journal titles and newspapers should be capitalized (e.g., *The Canadian Journal of Occupational Therapy*; *The Edmonton Journal*).

- For works that are not journals (books, articles, web pages, etc.), only the following should be capitalized: the first letter of the first word of a title; the first letter of the first word following a colon or a dash in the title; proper nouns (e.g., *Canadian nursing: Issues and perspectives*; Crunch time for public health care in Quebec).

| BOX 2.11 | Sample List of References |

References

Adinoff, A. (August 2002). Quality of care and outcomes of adults with asthma treated by specialists and generalists in managed care. *Pediatrics 110* (2). 454. Retrieved from Health Source Nursing Academic.

Barnes, P.J. (2003). New concepts in chronic obstructive pulmonary disease. *Annual Review of Medicine*, 54, 113–130.

Breathe easy: Good nutrition can help keep your lungs healthy. (June 2003). *Environmental Nutrition 26* (6). Retrieved April 22, 2009, from AltHealthWatch.

Grimes, GC., Manning, J.L., Patel, P., Via, M.R. (2007). Medication for COPD: A review of effectiveness. *American Family Physician 76* (8), 1141–1147.

Lee, T.A., Weaver, F.M., & Weiss, K.B. (January 2007). Impact of pneumococcal vaccination on pneumonia rates in patients with COPD and asthma. *JGIM: Journal of General Internal Medicine 22* (1). 62–67.

Moore, W.C. (May 15, 2009). Update in asthma 2008. *American Journal of Respiratory and Critical Care Medicine 179* (10). 869–875. Retrieved from Health Source Nursing Academic.

Public Health Agency of Canada. (May, 2006). Asthma. *It's your health*. Retrieved April 25, 2009, from http://www.hc-sc.gc.ca/hl-vs/iyh-vsv/diseases-maladies/asthm-eng.php

Stockley, R.A., Rennard, S., Rabe, K, & Celli, B. (2007). Chronic obstructive pulmonary disease. New Jersey: Wiley-Blackwell.

1. Prepare a list of at least five references in APA style for the sources found in the researching exercise on p. 38.
2. Take five books off your bookshelf and prepare a list of references for them.

PLAGIARISM

Every institution has its own definition of and official policy for dealing with plagiarism. Generally, though, plagiarism is understood as the act of knowingly submitting someone else's work as your own. To avoid plagiarism, you must acknowledge the sources of any ideas, words, or phrases that you use in your writing.

What is the difference between summarizing or paraphrasing and plagiarizing?

A summary or paraphrase of someone else's work includes a citation. Without the citation or mention of the original's author, it is plagiarism and is punishable by academic penalty.

Let's look at three different ways to incorporate a source into your writing:

Original

Sometimes, humans and animals can pass strains of flu back and forth to one another through direct close contact. When a swine influenza virus does affect a human, there is also a risk that the animal influenza can mutate and then spread directly between humans. More investigation is needed on how easily the virus spreads between people, but it is believed that it is spread the same way as regular seasonal influenza. Influenza and other respiratory infections are transmitted from person to person when germs enter the nose and/or throat.

Source: Public Health Agency of Canada. Fact Sheet H1N1 Flu Virus (Human Swine Flu, 2009). Retrieved, June 21, 2009, from http://www.phac-aspc.gc.ca/alert-alerte/swine-porcine/fs-fr_swine-eng.php

Version #1

It is possible for humans and animals to pass the flu to one another through direct contact. When a human contracts the swine flu virus, the animal influenza can mutate and spread directly between humans. There needs to be more research done into how easily the virus spreads between people, but it is believed that it is spread when germs enter the nose or throat, the same way as the regular flu.

Do you think this is plagiarism? Let's look at the two passages sentence by sentence:

Original: Sometimes, humans and animals can pass strains of flu back and forth to one another through direct close contact.

Version #1: It is possible for humans and animals to pass the flu to one another through direct contact.

Original: When a swine influenza virus does affect a human, there is also a risk that the animal influenza can mutate and then spread directly between humans.

Version #1: When a human contracts the swine flu virus, the animal influenza can mutate and spread directly between humans.

Original: More investigation is needed on how easily the virus spreads between people, but it is believed that it is spread the same way as regular seasonal influenza. Influenza and other respiratory infections are transmitted from person to person when germs enter the nose and/or throat.

Version #1: There needs to be more research done into how easily the virus spreads between people, but it is believed that it is spread when germs enter the nose or throat, the same way as the regular flu.

Is there a significant difference between the original and Version #1? Where does the information in Version #1 come from? If a student were to include these sentences in an essay or report, would they represent that student's original thought? Remember, you must cite anything in your writing that comes from somewhere else, even if the words have been changed.

Version #1 is an example of plagiarism. A student handing it in would receive a grade of 0 and may face further academic penalty.

The student could have avoided plagiarism by referring the source of the material, as seen in Version #2, below. Keep in mind that the source needs to be given every time paraphrased material is used.

Version #2

According to the Public Health Agency of Canada's *Fact Sheet for the H1N1 Flu Virus* (2009), it is possible for humans and animals to pass strains of influenza to one another. It is also possible for animal influenza to mutate and then pass from human to human. While more investigation is needed to determine how H1N1 is spread among humans, it is believed that, as with regular seasonal influenza, it is spread through germs entering the nose and/or throat.

Version #2 is a paraphrase; while the ideas come from somewhere else, the student has changed the wording and the order of the ideas. This is not plagiarism. When the exact wording of the original is used, use quotation marks, as in Version # 3, below.

Version #3

According to the Public Health Agency of Canada's *Fact Sheet for the H1N1 Flu Virus* (2009), it is possible for humans and animals to pass strains of influenza to one another. It is also possible for animal influenza to mutate and then pass from human to human. "There needs to be more research done into how easily the virus spreads between people, but it is believed that it is spread when germs enter the nose or throat, the same way as the regular flu" (*Fact Sheet*).

Why is plagiarism wrong?

Plagiarism is fraud. By copying someone's ideas and passing them off as your own, you are cheating that person out of his or her intellectual property. You are also demonstrating that you are unable to do the work required for the assigned task and that you lack the ability to think for yourself. Plagiarism can be dangerous in health-related fields; if you prepare a report using data you have hastily copied without checking, you may be spreading false information which may harm patients' health. Finally, you are leaving yourself open to legal action and limiting your employment possibilities.

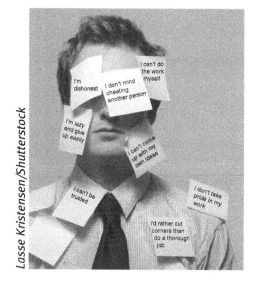

I'm dishonest

I don't mind cheating another person

I can't do the work myself

I'm lazy and give up easily

I can't come up with my own ideas

I'd rather cut corners than do a thorough job

I don't take pride in my work

I can't be trusted

Lasse Kristensen/Shutterstock

What does plagiarism say about you?

SAMPLE STUDENT APA REPORT

In the sample student report that follows (Box 2.12), excerpts from a much longer report have been used to model many of the APA formalities introduced in this chapter. Specifically, the model paper demonstrates proper formatting of the following key sections: title page, Abstract, tables, and figures sections as well as the References page. Additionally, the sample text pages model correct APA style headings and block quotation formatting as well as figure and table captioning.

BOX 2.12 | **Sample Student Report**

Running head: THE CAUSES OF HEARING LOSS

> The running head appears only on the title page.

The Causes of Hearing Loss

Erlinda S. Taruc

Humber College

> The report title, author, and institution should be double-spaced and centred on the title page.

Source: Courtesy of Erlinda Taruc.

The page header is placed one inch from the top of the page and flush left.

The Abstract should not exceed 120 words in length. It should summarize the main points of your research. The Abstract should be written in block format (it is not indented).

Abstract

Hearing is a sense through which a person experiences the world he or she lives in. Reduction or complete loss of sensitivity to sound, however, can greatly affect and limit a person's participation in daily activities. Consequently, knowing the source of one's hearing problem is essential to one's well being. Causes of hearing loss vary and are often dependant on time of onset, severity and age. When attempting to categorize the causes of hearing loss, the origins of the loss must be taken into consideration. This informative report explains causes of hearing loss originating from external, middle, or inner ear damage . Hearing loss that originates in these three areas is classified as conductive, sensorineural, or mixed.

Conductive Hearing Loss (CHL)

This is a Level 1 APA heading. Text should be bolded, centred, and use standard capitalization.

Hearing disorders that affect the outer and middle ear are termed conductive hearing loss. CHL arises when a blockage, physical defect, or damage to these structures prevents sound from reaching the inner ear. The external auditory canal may be blocked, the three tiny bones of the middle ear may fail to conduct sound to the cochlea, or the eardrum may fail to vibrate in response to sound. These problems may be corrected by medical or surgical interventions. (Burkey, 2003). Figure 1 illustrates an overview of the human ear.

Causes of Conductive Hearing Loss

This is a Level 2 APA heading. Text should be flush left, bolded, and use standard capitalization.

Some of the possible causes of conductive hearing loss include a lodged object in the ear canal, excessive amount of wax blocking the ear canal, infection in the outer or middle ear cavity, puncturing of the eardrum, disconnection of the middle ear bones, and deformity of the outer or middle ear.

Foreign bodies in the external auditory canal. Children sometimes push small bits and pieces, such as pebbles, bugs, beads, toy parts, cereals, and other food particles into their ear canals. The obstruction can result in discomfort, aches, infection, or hearing loss (Cole & Flexer, 2007).

This is a Level 3 APA heading. Text should be lowercase, bolded, and indented. A Level 3 heading must be followed by a period.

Cerumen or earwax impaction. This condition occurs when there is an excessive amount of earwax or cerumen that blocks the ear canal. Cerumen is a typical body secretion found along the skin of the ear canal of the outer ear. Earwax protects the auditory canal by discouraging dust and other air borne particles from entering and getting too deep into the eventually lead to hearing impairment (Isaacson & Vora, 2003). Marcincuk and Roland (2002) further elaborate:

Quotes longer than 40 words are set off as block quotations. Notice, in block quotes, that the final period is placed before the bracketed source information.

> Exostoses occur when the external canal is repeatedly exposed to cold air or water. Cold exposure irritates the periosteum [connective tissue membrane that surrounds all bones except those at joints] and stimulates bony growth ... Osteomas are benign neoplasms [tumors] of the bone. They are less common than exostoses and are usually single and unilateral [hearing loss in one ear]. (p. 48)

Sensorineural Hearing Loss (SNHL)

When a hearing loss results from disorders in the inner ear, it is referred to as sensorineural hearing loss. The damage is usually in the cochlea, which contains numerous microscopic sensory receptors called hair cells. These inner hair cells convert sound vibrations into electrical signals that travel as nerve impulses to the brain, where their meanings are processed and interpreted. Problems in the auditory nerves, which send sound to the brain, also contribute to SNHL (Burkey, 2003). Table 1 defines various degrees of hearing loss including sensorineural loss.

Accordingly, Tang, Montemayor, and Pereira (2006) state, "Many hearing disorders involve irreversible damage to hair cells and their associated nerves and result in permanent hearing impairment ... known as sensorineural hearing loss" (p. 525). SNHL can affect the clarity of hearing and volume of sound, so even if sound is loud enough to be perceived, substantial sound distortion can occur which results in difficulty understanding speech (Hewitt & Wareing, 2006).

References

Burkey, J.M. (2003). *Overcoming hearing aid fears: The road to better hearing*. New Jersey: Rutgers.

Canadian Academy of Audiology (2006). The ear [figure]. In *How do we hear*. Retrieved Mar ch 29, 2008, from http://www.canadianaudiology.ca/consumers/children/index.html.

Canadian Hearing Instrument Practioners Society. Degree of hearing loss [table]. In *Canadian consumer guide to hearing loss and hearing aids* (4). Retrieved April 1, 2008, from hearCanada.com/Consumers/Consumer-Guide.Pdf.

Cole, E.B., & Flexer, C. (2007). *Children with hearing loss: Developing listening and talking*. San Diego: Plural.

Isaacson, J., & Vora, N. (2003, September 15). Differential diagnosis and treatment of hearing loss. *American Family Physician, 68*(6), 1125–1132.

Marcincuk, M., & Roland, P. (2002, April). Understanding the causes and providing appropriate treatment. *Geriatrics, 57*(4), 44.

Miller, M., & Schein, J. (2005, July). Selected complex auditory disorders. *Journal of Rehabilitation Research & Development, 42*, 1–8.

Newton, V., & Vallely, P. (Eds.). (2006). *Infection and hearing impairment*. West Sussex: Whurr.

Subha, S., & Raman, R. (2006). Role of impacted cerumen in hearing loss. *ENT: Ear, Nose & Throat Journal, 85*(10), 650–653.

Tang, L., Montemayor, C., & Pereira, F. (2006, September). Sensorineural hearing loss: Potential therapies and gene targets for drug development. *IUBMB Life, 58*(9), 525–530.

The References list appears after the body of the report and is double-spaced. Entries are alphabetized according to the author's surname or, in the absence of an author, the first word of the source's title.

References are formatted using a hanging indent: the first lines of entries begin at the margin and second and subsequent lines are indented half an inch from the left margin. All sources cited in your report must be listed on the References page.

Table 1.
Degree of Hearing Loss

Place tables after the References section. Tables should be captioned as shown. Complete table captioning instructions are provided on pp. 52 .

Hearing Threshold	Description of Hearing
0 dB	Perfect
1 – 25 dB	Normal
26 – 40 dB	Mild Loss
41 – 55 dB	Moderate Loss
56 – 80 dB	Severe Loss
81+ dB	Profound Loss

Note: Table adapted from *Canadian Consumer Guide to Hearing Loss and Hearing Aids*, p. 4.

Figure Captions

Figure 1. **The anatomy of the human ear.**

> Place figure captions on a separate page and format as shown. Complete figure captioning instructions are provided on pp. 52.

Each figure is placed on a separate page immediately following the Figure Captions page.

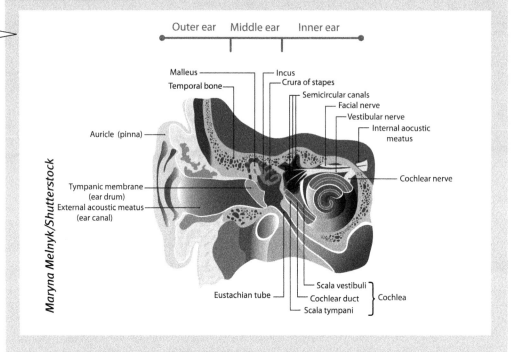

Note: Figure taken from *Canadian Academy of Audiology* website, 2006.

CHARACTERISTICS OF GOOD ACADEMIC WRITING

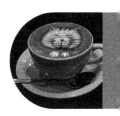

Write in CLEAR language. For summaries and critical analyses, do not "translate" the original document word for word with a thesaurus; you will end up with something that does not make sense. For all academic documents, avoid technical jargon and use words that you are familiar with. Don't try to sound "smart"—it always backfires!

Be OBJECTIVE. Any opinions expressed in academic writing must be backed up by facts. Don't rely on your "feelings" or "beliefs." Use the first-person singular ("I") sparingly, and avoid it completely in summaries and academic reports.

Academic writing should be CONCISE. Include the necessary information, but edit out unnecessary details, digressions, or information that does not directly support your thesis or serve the purpose of the document.

Academic writing should be ORGANIZED according to the guidelines for the specific type of document. Whichever method of organization you use, make sure that the ideas proceed logically. Ask a classmate or friend to read through your essay, report, summary, or analysis to ensure that the document is easy to follow.

Provide the reader with ACCURATE information; do your research carefully and double-check facts when possible.

As always, proofread all written documents to ensure CORRECT grammar, spelling, and punctuation. A grammatical error or confused word can undermine your credibility; your reader may assume that you are careless and therefore not a reliable source of information.

Be sure that your writing is AUDIENCE-APPROPRIATE; if it is aimed at a general audience, do not use overly technical or specialized vocabulary. Define any unfamiliar terms.

Academic writing must be THOROUGH. In a summary or analysis, do not miss any of the original's main points. In an essay or report, cover all sides of an argument and/or provide all relevant information. Be sure to document all sources used.

CHAPTER 3

WRITING IN
A PROFESSIONAL SETTING

At the end of this chapter, you should be able to:

- produce effective resumés and cover letters
- review sample resumés and cover letters to determine their strengths and weaknesses
- write professional emails in the health care workplace
- understand how to write narrative progress notes and structured progress notes (SOAP, DAR, PIE)
- determine the advantages and disadvantages of both the structured and the unstructured progress note
- recognize the influence of technology in medical documentation and record-keeping.

INTRODUCTION

Previous chapters prepared you to meet the writing demands of your college or university health sciences program. Now it is time to prepare you for what you have strived so hard for: being successful in the health care workplace.

Graduation from college or university followed by entrance into the workplace is an exciting time in most people's lives. After the financial and time investments of a postsecondary education, it is time to reap the rewards of the educational investment that you have made. There is nothing worse than putting effort and discipline into a college or university degree only to find that you cannot secure that perfect job after graduation.

To reduce the chances of this occurring, the first step in successfully transitioning from school to workplace is the creation of an effective resumé and cover letter that will demonstrate to potential employers why you are the best candidate for the health care job that interests you. This is exactly what you will learn to do at the outset of this chapter.

Then, once you have landed your desired health care job, (because of your top-notch resumé), you will need to demonstrate on a daily basis that you can meet the writing demands of your particular profession. The section on professional correspondence in this chapter guides you toward this goal by providing some useful tips on presenting yourself professionally and diplomatically in your everyday written communication.

Finally, this chapter concludes by introducing you to the most common ways that health care professionals like nurses, paramedics, occupational therapists, and physiotherapists document and monitor patient health. To this end, the final section of this chapter provides a basic overview of the progress note, structured and unstructured, as well as the advantages and disadvantages of computerized documentation systems.

RESUMÉS AND COVER LETTERS

While you will write many important documents in your professional life, the cover letter and resumé are the two documents that will open up professional doors for you. Many people underestimate the importance of these documents. Your cover letter and resumé inform prospective employers about more than just your education and experience: they demonstrate your attention to detail and ability to communicate clearly—crucial skills in the allied health professions.

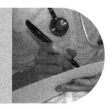

I was hiring a pharmacy assistant and I received many resumés from qualified applicants. One recent college graduate had the required education and experience; however, he misspelled several words—including "pharmacy" and the name of his college—on his resumé. In my business, one tiny mistake can have tragic consequences; we can't afford to hire someone who is careless. This applicant did not get the job.

—Pharmacist, Winnipeg, MB

The Goals of Your Resumé and Cover Letter

1. Grab the reader's attention.

   DO … use catchy headings that are relevant to the position you are applying for
   DO … use a professional and consistent layout
   DO … make it visually appealing
   DON'T … use coloured paper or ink

2. Capture the reader's interest.

   DO … clearly identify your key traits
   DO … highlight skills and experiences that are relevant for the position
   DO … show why you would be an asset to the organization
   DON'T … lie, or even exaggerate

3. Encourage the reader to contact you.

   DO … offer to provide more information, such as work samples and ideas
   DO … ask for an interview
   DO … provide your phone number and email address
   DON'T … provide unprofessional email addresses—sexyvixen@hotmail.com
   does not fit the image of a competent health care professional!

The Resumé

Your resumé provides your prospective employer with a summary of your skills, qualities, and experience. Frequently, employers receive more than one hundred applications for a single position; therefore, they may look at each resumé for less than a minute. How can you make a positive impression and become one of the very few selected for an interview?

Tips for Writing Your Resumé

1. Use titles or headings that match the jobs you want.

   – If applying for a nursing position, you may choose to use the heading "Nursing Qualifications."

2. Create a design that attracts attention and identifies your key attributes.

   – Most resumés include the following sections: Skills/Qualifications; Employment Experience; Education. However, you may want to add Academic Accomplishments or Personal Attributes, depending on your strongest qualities. Ask yourself what sets you apart from other applicants. Put that information first.

3. Customize your resumé to every job.

   – Emphasize the skills and experience that are suited to the particular job you are applying for. List skills in order of relevance.

4. Use key words from the job advertisement.

   – Employers carefully select the wording of an advertisement to reflect the qualities that they see as important. Read the ad carefully, and use the same key words (for example, "collaborate with…," "assess extent of…," "document and record…").

5. Use "accomplishment words" (see Box 3.1).

   – These words indicate that you have made significant contributions to your previous workplaces or educational institutions.

BOX 3.1	**Accomplishment Words**	
achieved	improved	remodelled
activated	increased	reorganized
addressed	initiated	represented
administered	launched	researched
built	led	restructured
conducted	motivated	shaped
consulted	operated	solved
created	organized	stimulated
demonstrated	overhauled	strengthened
developed	performed	supervised
enabled	planned	trained
engineered	prepared	upgraded
facilitated	presented	worked
guided	produced	wrote
identified	recommended	
implemented	reduced	

Matthew Lui

3607 19th St. SE
Calgary AB
T5A 0B4
(403) 555-5555
Email: mattlui@hotmail.com

PROFESSIONAL QUALIFICATIONS

- Familiar with ProPharm and Kroll systems
- Proficient in Microsoft Office 2007
- Able to learn new procedures very quickly
- Honest and reliable individual who enjoys working with people

Professional Qualifications section highlights skills and qualities relevant to the position applied for.

EDUCATION

Pharmacy Technician Diploma   April 2008

Bow Valley College, Calgary AB

WORK EXPERIENCE

Pharmacy Assistant (Co-op)   Jan 2006–April 2007

- Checked invoices to ensure accuracy of client information
- Assisted pharmacist with dispensing prescriptions
- Maintained inventory, checked expired drugs

Work Experience section uses accomplishment words (*checked, assisted, maintained, consulted, provided, handled,* and *referred*) to highlight the applicant's positive impact on past places of employment.

Cashier   Jan 2003–Dec 2003

Millerdale Pharmacy, Red Deer AB

- Consulted with customers to determine their needs and provide suggestions
- Provided excellent customer service and product knowledge
- Handled and referred customer inquiries

REFERENCES AVAILABLE UPON REQUEST

Source: Adapted from documents provided by Humber College's Career Services

Anna Petersen

60 Clipper Road, #706
Toronto, ON M2J 4E2
(416) 497-3294
Email: apetersen@hotmail.com

The Personal Profile section uses action words (*communicates, brings, assists,* and *works*). Note that these words are all grammatically parallel (in the same grammatical form), as well.

OBJECTIVE

To be an active member of a multidisciplinary team in a challenging setting, and to provide efficient, quality, family-centred care to clients.

PERSONAL PROFILE

- Communicates and interacts effectively with individuals on all levels.
- Brings enthusiasm and devotion to encourage a client-oriented environment.
- Assists staff, clients, and supervisors in identifying and resolving problems.
- Works well with others toward achieving team goals or alone as an individual.

RELEVANT PROFESSIONAL EXPERIENCE

Emergency Services–Registered Nurse	Toronto, Ont.
Closing the Gap Healthcare Group	March 2008–Present
Emergency Services–Registered Nurse	Toronto, Ont.
SRT MED-STAFF	December 2006–March 2008
Emergency Services–Registered Nurse	Toronto, Ont.
St. Joseph's Health Centre	January 2006–December 2006

EDUCATION

Bachelor of Science with Honours – Nursing	2000–2005
York University/Seneca College	
Social Service Worker – Gerontology	1999–2000
Seneca College of Applied Arts & Technology	
Emergency First Aid – Level C and CPR Certified	

Volunteer experience shows that the applicant is caring and compassionate, and values experience over money.

VOLUNTEER EXPERIENCE

Private Tutor	2000–2009
Multiple Sclerosis Society	2005–2008
Heart & Stroke Foundation	2005–2008

REFERENCES AVAILABLE UPON REQUEST

The Cover Letter

Never discount the importance of the cover letter—it is the basis for your reader's first impression of you. A cover letter shouldn't just summarize your resumé; it should draw the reader's attention to your strengths, highlighting those qualities that set you apart from the competition.

The Parts of a Cover Letter

1. Introduction

    - Tell the reader what position you are applying for and where you saw the advertisement.
    - Briefly explain why you want to work for this organization and why you want this specific position.

2. Body

    - Briefly outline your best qualities and your most relevant skills for the job.
    - State how your skills would benefit the company.

3. Conclusion

    - Clearly ask for an interview. Provide contact information.

Tips for Writing Your Cover Letter

1. Include your data and the recipient's data at the top of the page

    - Include your name, address, phone number(s), email address.
    - Include the recipient's work title, address, and name (if available). If you do not know the recipient's name, use the title given in the advertisement. "Dear Human Resources" or "Dear Hiring Manager" is preferable to "To Whom it May Concern."

2. Keep it simple and direct

    - Employers often receive hundreds of applications for one job opening; you have about 30 seconds to get your message across.
    - A cover letter should fit on one page.

3. Do not omit necessary information

    - Include all information specifically requested, such as availability and salary expectations.

4. Proofread carefully and read out loud to check style and flow

    - A single error can cause the reader to reject your application.

5. Make your letter a reflection of you

- – Customize your letter to fit each position.
- – Avoid clichés ("I'm a people person").
- – Do not make any claims that you cannot back up with actions.

One of the core values of our health care organization is to "treat everyone with respect and dignity." As you know, Toronto is a multicultural city, and staff must work with colleagues and patients of different ethnicities. It is important that candidates understand and respect diversity. I've seen some candidates write standard blanket statements that they "work well with and get along with other people." In one interview, one of the questions I asked was, "What type of people do you not *like to work with?" The candidate looked carefully around the room to make sure no one was around, and very quietly said to me, "Well, to be honest with you, I don't like to work too much with black people." Needless to say, I was in shock, and this closed the door to any job opportunities for this person. Moral of the story: Understand the mission, vision, and values of the organization to which you are applying. Ensure that your cover letter and resumé truly and accurately reflect who you are and align with the culture of that organization. Don't say things you don't mean, as the truth will likely come out in the interview when you least expect it.*

—Supervisor, University Health Network, Toronto, ON

Jasmeet Singh

76-3468 Drummond Street
Montreal, Quebec
H3G 1Y4
514-842-5293
singhj@gmail.com

March 31st, 2009.

Dear Hiring Manager,

It is with great interest and enthusiasm that I am applying for the position of Case Manager, which was advertised in the *Globe and Mail* on Wednesday, June 10, 2009. This is a position in which my three years of relevant nursing experience can have an immediate and positive impact.

Throughout my clinical placement, I have successfully increased productivity and efficiency and have clearly demonstrated my ability to manage multiple projects and tasks concurrently with excellent follow-through and attention to quality.

I have illustrated exceptional communication and leadership skills through my work with individuals at all levels, and have been highly effective in establishing rapport with clients, co-workers, and management.

You will benefit from my ability to foster a desired sense of comfort and deliver superior client-centered care. I have consistently displayed strong interpersonal skills and a genuine interest in meeting the needs of individuals, families, and the community at large.

I am enthusiastic and eager about working in a role that is ideally suited to my personal qualities and professional skills. An interview will provide us with an opportunity to discuss our needs and demonstrate further how I can add great value to your organization. I look forward to hearing from you.

Sincerely,

Jasmeet Singh

The letter opens by demonstrating the applicant's enthusiasm, identifying which position is being applied for and where it was advertised, and highlighting the qualities and experiences that make the applicant well-suited for the job.

This shows the impact that the applicant has had on his former place of work and implies that he can make the same improvements in his next job.

This shows that he communicates well with others and is a team player. Note the use of the word "effective."

Here, the applicant clearly outlines the benefits for the entire organization.

The applicant closes by reiterating his enthusiasm, telling the reader why he wants the position, and showing why he is right for the position. He then requests an interview, suggesting that he wants the opportunity to prove that he is the right person for the job.

1. Find an advertisement for a job in your chosen field and tailor your resumé for it, using the suggestions from this chapter. Write a cover letter to accompany it. Don't forget to proofread both very carefully. Exchange with a classmate and critique each other's letter and resumé as if you were an employer.

PROFESSIONAL E-CORRESPONDENCE

Electronic correspondence has replaced letters in many circumstances. There are many benefits to email: it reduces response time, it saves paper, and it provides an electronic record of your correspondence.

However, many people fail to distinguish between casual and professional emails, which can lead to misunderstandings and loss of credibility. There are several things to keep in mind when writing emails in an academic or professional setting.

Tips for Writing Professional Emails

1. Provide a clear and specific subject heading.

    – This prevents emails from being rejected as spam and allows the recipient to prioritize his/her messages.
    – Example: Revised August Schedule for Floor Three Nurses

2. Begin your email with a proper greeting, just as you would in a written letter.

    – This shows respect for the recipient and establishes a formal tone.
    – Example: Dear Dr. Singh; Dear Kevin; Dear Professor Sinopoli.
    – Be sure to check the spelling of names.

3. Identify yourself.

    – Always sign your name.
    – When writing to a teacher, include your full name and course/section number.
    – When writing to a professional colleague, include your job title and department or division.

4. Follow the standards of academic or professional writing.

    – Write in complete, grammatically correct sentences.
    – Use a professional font (e.g., Times Roman, Arial), size, and colour.
    – Use standard spelling, punctuation, and capitalization.

5. Keep the email brief.

- The message should fit on one screen.
- Each email should be limited to one subject. Do not confuse your reader by attempting to deal with multiple issues in one email.

6. Pause before sending.

- Check for spelling, punctuation, and grammar errors
- Ask yourself if the content of your email is appropriate. If your boss were to see it, what would his or her reaction be?

7. Use a serious, professional tone.

- Jokes and sarcasm may be misinterpreted as rude and/or insulting.

Raising or Responding to Sensitive Issues in an Email

While face-to-face communication is ideal for discussing sensitive issues (requests, complaints, conflicts, and so on), sometimes an email is necessary to either request a meeting, follow up on an earlier conversation, or respond to a situation. In such cases, follow these guidelines:

1. Briefly state the history and context of the issue.

2. Outline any actions you have taken to resolve the issue.

3. Give reasons that it is necessary for this issue to be resolved quickly.

4. Suggest possible solutions.

5. If the issue is particularly complicated or sensitive, or if nothing is resolved after a few emails, request a face-to-face meeting.

6. Keep your tone neutral. Avoid sounding aggressive, threatening, or defensive.

7. If you are angry about the issue, compose the email and then wait a day before sending. Re-read your message carefully to avoid saying anything you could regret later.

8. Check grammar, spelling, and punctuation carefully.

To: lawrence_chan@brandonu.ca
From: dylan_cornacchia@brandon.ca

Subject: Dylan Cornacchia, Student # 9945023

Dear Professor Chan,

I am a student in your section of Nursing Foundations II that meets Tuesdays and Thursdays.

The course outline indicates that we have a test scheduled for Tuesday, March 10. I have a medical condition that requires frequent specialists' appointments, and there is an appointment scheduled for the same time as the test. I tried to reschedule the appointment, but there is a three-month waiting period.

My doctor's office is sending me a note showing that I do have an appointment at that time. I will give it to you when I receive it.

Is it possible for me to write the test on an earlier or later date? Please let me know what I can do to avoid losing the marks for this test. If you would like to discuss this issue in person, I can meet you during your office hours next week.

Best,

Dylan Cornacchia

To: David Bernstein <david_bernstein@ssc.ca>
From: Florence Nguyen <Florence_nguyen@ssc.ca>

Subject: Violet Abela

Dear Mr. Bernstein

From our brief conversation this morning, I understand that you received a phone call from Mrs. Symington, expressing her dissatisfaction with the treatment her mother (Ms. Violet Abela) is receiving.

I have been working with Ms. Abela for three weeks now, and I am confident that I have followed protocol and behaved professionally. In addition, I have noticed a marked improvement in Ms. Abela's range of motion.

I understand that Mrs. Symington has raised similar complaints over the three months her mother has been a resident here. The satisfaction of our clients and their families is very important to me. I would be happy if we could meet soon to discuss this further.

Regards,

Florence Nguyen
OTA
Sunnyside Seniors' Centre

> The writer begins with a formal salutation, as in a letter. If you are on friendly terms with the recipient, use his or her first name, but be professional.

> The context of the situation is clearly stated. If your email is in response to an earlier conversation or correspondence, indicate this.

> The writer provides her opinion of the situation in a clear, non-defensive manner.

> The writer gives more context, and emphasizes her desire to reach a solution. She ends with a request for a face-to-face meeting.

> The letter concludes respectfully ("regards") and includes the writer's full name and position.

1. Rewrite the following email, to make it more appropriate and effective.

   To: brian.simpson@senecac.on.ca

   From: prettygirl@hotmail.com

   Subject: Just a reminder

   Hey Sir, I was wondering if it were possible to boost my final mark by 3%. I'm sort 3% to receive the scholarship of $1000. At this point i will have to go to summer school just to get 3%. PLEASE PLEASE PLEASE PLEASE i tried me hardest. If you can, it would mean a lot to me and will also assist in my finical situation. I will take anything you can give if possible. Thanks! Amanpreet ☺

2. You have been working as a health care professional in a probationary capacity for six months. This is your first job in the field. While your six-month performance evaluation says you are enthusiastic and devoted, it also states that you are, on occasion, insufficiently focused on your job and sometimes seem to be lost. Furthermore, you have been late to work twice in the past three months. Finally, your supervisor says you sometimes lack patience.

   While flawless performance evaluations are not expected—especially after only six months—you know that this could affect your chances of getting hired back at the end of a year.

   Write an email to your boss, offering your interpretation of the evaluation and trying to convince him or her that you are indeed a capable employee. Make up any necessary details, including names and dates.

CHARACTERISTICS OF GOOD PROFESSIONAL WRITING

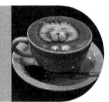

Communicate your message in CLEAR language. Professional writing should be direct and to-the-point; if the reader doesn't know what you are trying to say, he or she will probably not bother reading further. If you are asking that action be taken, be sure to state precisely what the desired outcome is.

When providing information about an incident or issue, be sure to remain OBJECTIVE. Do not resort to accusations or name-calling. State the facts, and leave the emotions out.

Health care professionals are busy; therefore, professional correspondence should be CONCISE. Keep emails to one screen-length. Keep resumés and letters to one page.

Present your information in an ORGANIZED manner. In letters and emails, begin with a greeting, followed by your reason for writing, a summary of the issue, a proposed solution, and a call for action.

Check your facts to ensure that you are presenting an ACCURATE picture of the situation. Facts can be checked, so never stretch the truth in a resumé, letter, or email.

Always proofread professional correspondence to ensure that it is grammatically CORRECT. Errors can reduce your credibility in the eyes of your employer, colleagues, or professor.

Adopt an AUDIENCE-APPROPRIATE tone. Avoid abbreviations (lol) and emoticons (☺).

Provide a THOROUGH picture of whatever you are presenting, whether it be a patient's history, an on-the-job conflict, or your own employment history. Include all necessary information, including dates, quantities, and the like. If information is too sensitive to include in an email, request an appointment to speak in person.

DOCUMENTATION SYSTEMS IN HEALTH CARE FACILITIES

Now that you have secured that desired health care job through the creation of a proper cover letter and resumé, it is time to look at the specific types of writing you will be doing once you start working with actual patients.

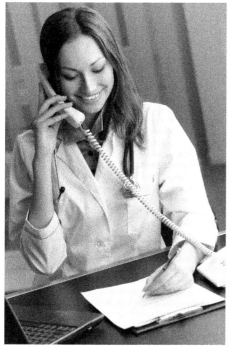

vgstudio/Shutterstock

THE PROGRESS NOTE

There are many different ways of documenting a patient's condition throughout the caregiving process and the type of documentation required will depend on your health care role as well as on the requirements of the facility where you work. One of the most important documents in the health care workplace is the progress note. A **progress note** is a document which records, tracks, and monitors a patient's health status. While formats and styles of progress notes vary, health care professionals like doctors, nurses, psychiatrists, and personal support workers are all responsible for carefully documenting observations and assessments of their patients from the point of admission through to the point of discharge. And in acute care facilities, health care workers are required to frequently update a patient's health status. So, with all the writing that is required in a health care institution, it is a good idea to get into good writing habits now. Below, you will be introduced to two common types of progress notes: the narrative note and the structured note (SOAP, SOAPIE, SOAPIER, DAR, PIE).

The Narrative Note

Traditionally, narrative notes that read like mini-stories were the main way that health care providers documented patient care. Today, while the majority of health care facilities seem to prefer more structured patient notes, some institutions still require that a patient's health be updated using the narrative note.

Advantages of the narrative note:

- Narrative charting is easy to learn. There are no complicated formulas or formatting procedures to remember.
- Because narrative charting does not require a lot in terms of format and style, it is flexible and adaptable to various facilities.
- Narrative charting can be an effective way to convey health intentions and patient responses.
- The narrative format can help personalize the patient-caregiver relationship as the patient's health is not reduced to an acronym or formula.

Disadvantages of the narrative note:

- A lack of formatting requirements can lead to inconsistency in record-keeping, which may sacrifice quality of patient care.
- As a mini-story, this type of progress note can appear less scientific than some of the more structured formats like SOAP, PIE, and DAR and may encourage the incorporation of too much subjective detail.
- The narrative style can lead to "over-charting," particularly for new workers who need time to master how to distinguish essential detail from non-essential detail.
- Because of its lack of a fixed organizational structure, repetition of detail can result.
- It can be difficult for readers of the unstructured narrative note to find specific information quickly and effortlessly.

As you can see in the sample narrative note below, relevant patient information is presented as a mini-story.

Sample Narrative Note

June 26th, 2009 @ 0745:
Pt. was aware and alert this morning and oriented to time, place, and person.
Pt. observably distressed, tearful, and anxious. While discussing pt's needs, pt.
expressed anxiety and fear with regard to his current health experience. Stated
"I am so afraid of dying," and "It's my family that seems unable to let me go
and say goodbye." Discussed with pt. his fears of dying and proposed grief
counselling services as well as offered to call a family member for added support.
Pt. observably less anxious and distressed post-interview. Informs that current
plan of care and proposed services are satisfactory to his needs and that he does
not wish to see any relatives at present. VS otherwise consistent; BP 120/60,
HR 65 regular, O2 98% RA, RR 18, T-36.9 tympanic. Skin pink, warm, and
dry. Chest clear, abdomen soft, no tenderness. IV in situ and infusing well NS at
100cc/hr. At present no acute concerns. Will follow through with proposed plan
of care and monitor ongoing. Call bell within reach. Winter Eve Hill RN

Source: Courtesy of Winter Eve Hill.

The Structured Note (SOAP, SOAPIE, and SOAPIER)

Structured progress notes can be organized in many different ways, as you will see.
Despite differences in formatting and organization of the structured progress note, the
categories of focus are similar and include variations on the following themes: problem,
assessment, intervention, and evaluation. Workplaces have different preferences when
it comes to charting formalities, so it is best to check with your workplace to see what
method of documentation they prefer.

Advantages of the structured note:

* Acronyms like SOAP, PIE, and DAR are easy to remember and are effective ways
  of setting up and organizing patient information.
* As caregivers rely on the same structure to create their notes, there is consistency
  in the documentation process.
* Consistent and organized recording of relevant information can result in better
  communication and decreased levels of frustration.
* Other team members can easily locate useful and relevant patient data because of
  the clearly defined and consistently ordered categories of information.

Disadvantages of the structured note:

* There are concerns that the formulaic nature of structured progress notes does not
  allow for a comprehensive account of the patient's progress.
* Sometimes additional or supplementary notes may be required for important
  information that does not fit into any of the SOAP, DAR, or PIE formulas.
* Training is required for health care professionals to properly understand and
  correctly use structured progress notes.

The SOAP Note

S = subjective

> Subjective detail includes what the patient and his or her caregivers tell you about the symptoms that are of concern. Recording a patient's exact words is preferred to paraphrasing.

O = objective

> Objective data includes the health care provider's observation of the patient (body language, affect) as well as records vital signs, test results and medications given.

A = assessment

> The assessment of the patient's condition is based on an evaluation of both subjective and objective data.

P = plan

> Based on the assessment, a treatment plan is documented. The treatment plan should include both long-term and short-term measures.

Sometimes facilities require an extension of the SOAP format. You may be asked to use SOAPIE or SOAPIER.

I = intervention

> This section can be used to record a change in treatment plan.

E = evaluation

> Here, the treatment plan is evaluated for progress and effect.

R = revision

> Based on the outcome and evaluation of the treatment plan, revisions or recommendations might be necessary and are recorded here.

Sample SOAP Note

June 26, 2009 @ 0745:

S: "I am so afraid of dying. How will my family support themselves; how will I cope with the pain? I can't believe this is happening to me, and yet, strangely, I'm ready. It's my family that seems unable to let me go and say goodbye".

O: Pt. presents with observable anxiety and distress related to his current health experience. Pt. expresses his fears of death, and the pain that may be related to it, as well as his family's inability to let him go and accept that his life may be nearing the end.

A: Pt. afraid of death and dying and has anxiety related to his family's future as well as their inability to accept the possibility of his passing.

P: Grief counsellor called to bedside to assist and support both the pt. and his family during his current health experience. Care plan regarding pain management and pt's present needs discussed briefly with pt. Winter Eve Hill RN

Source: Courtesy of Winter Eve Hill.

The PIE Note

P = problem

This is similar to the subjective detail recorded in the SOAP note. The problem is the patient's reason for seeking help or assistance.

I = intervention

This is a record of how the patient's health concern was addressed. This might include the prescription of medication or a referral to a health specialist.

E = evaluation

Here the health care worker provides an evaluation of the effectiveness of the proposed intervention strategies.

Sample PIE Note

June 26, 2009 @ 1005:
P: Called to bedside. Pt. received in observable distress. C/o severe RLQ abdo pain, 8/10. Grimacing and writhing in bed, clutching abdomen.

I: 6mg Morphine with 50cc NS given via IV. Pt. Repositioned in bed.

E: Pt. states pain has decreased to 3/10, 15 mins post analgesia. Resting comfortably at present. Denies any further needs. Will monitor ongoing for therapeutic effect of pain management and administer analgesia as required. Winter Eve Hill RN

Source: Courtesy of Winter Eve Hill.

The DAR Note

D = data

In the DAR note, all subjective and objective data is recorded in the same section.

A = action

This is an account of the proposed care plan based on the assembled health data.

R = response

The patients' responses to the implemented interventions are recorded here.

Sample DAR Note

June 26, 2009 @ 0745:

D: Pt. received observably distressed. Expressed anxiety and fear with regard to his current health experience. Fearful of death and dying, and concerned that he may experience pain. Pt. expressed his anxiety and distress related to his family's future, and is concerned that they have not yet accepted his current health status, and the possibility of his passing.

A: Discussed with pt. his current plan of care, and discussed his potential needs for pain management and therapy. Called grief counsellor to bedside for both pt. and family support.

R: Pt. expressed a great deal of relief with regard to his current plan of care and pain management, as well as proposed services. Observably more comfortable and less anxious. Pt. denies any further needs at present; will evaluate therapeutic effect of pain management as well as supportive services ongoing throughout the day. Winter Eve Hill RN

Source: Courtesy of Winter Eve Hill.

CHARTING BY EXCEPTION

In the high stress and fast pace of the busy health care environment, the "no frills" approach to patient charting, known as charting by exception (CBE), is becoming an increasingly popular way to document patient progress. CBE requires that only significant or abnormal health occurrences are recorded, thereby eliminating lengthy and repetitive notes. In this type of charting, the caregiver uses tick charts or flow sheets to record abnormal activity.

Advantages of CBE:

- The time spent on the task of documenting a patient's health progress is significantly decreased by recording only abnormal activity.
- Tick and flow sheets eliminate the need for lengthy and time-consuming notes.
- Changes and concerns in a patient's health are easily spotted.
- CBE is usually done at the patient's bedside, allowing for immediate recording of data which may decrease documentation errors that result from delayed charting or charting after the fact.

Disadvantages of CBE:

- There is a concern that a comprehensive account of a patient's condition cannot be achieved by focusing only on the problematic.
- CBE requires an extensive repository of flow sheets customized to reflect the variety of medical experiences that health care workers encounter in a care facility.

- CBE appears to focus on obvious changes, potentially neglecting less obvious but nonetheless important changes.
- Sometimes CBE notes need to be supplemented with progress notes which detract from the goal of efficiency.
- The development of guidelines and standards of care required to use CBE is time-consuming.
- The caregiver has to demonstrate knowledge of established assessment guidelines in order to use CBE properly.
- Caregivers have to receive training and practice in CBE.

DOCUMENTATION AND THE COMPUTER

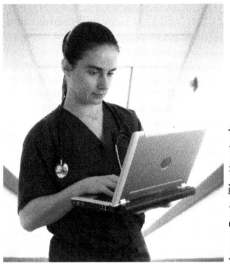

Ioana Drutu/Shutterstock

Practically all health care facilities today rely to some extent on computerized documentation systems. Computerized medical information systems allow the health care worker to access a wide range of important patient data by simply entering a personal access code or password.

Advantages of computerized documentation systems:

- Efficiency of documentation is increased, particularly if computers are placed at patients' bedsides for immediate recording of data.
- Basic computer fonts are much easier to read than handwritten notes.
- With electronic storage of information, medical data can be centralized.
- Clinical and statistical data can easily be calculated and retrieved.
- Computers have the capability of reducing some documentation errors as many current systems provide an alert message if patient data is entered incorrectly or not at all.

Disadvantages of computerized documentation systems:

- Medical records are private matters and computer systems raise questions about the confidentiality and security of such data.
- The assumption exists that health care workers will have the essential computer skills to succeed in an electronic environment.
- If technology used in a medical facility breaks down it has the potential to cause significant lapses in care as well as loss of valuable data—which could potentially be life-threatening.
- Electronic systems can be expensive to install and maintain.
- Standardized forms and databases raise the concern of whether individualization of patient care is compromised.
- Computerized documentation is dependent on the accuracy of information entered by the health care worker.
- The computer can aid in efficiency but does not provide the personal contact and connection that are central to the patient–caregiver relationship.

MEDICAL FORMS

Aside from potential charting duties, as a future health care provider you will be required to fill out numerous other forms based on your professional role and the requirements of the facility where you work. Whether your facility requires you to fill out forms electronically or by hand, when filling out medical forms in the workplace make sure you abide by the following rules:

- Be neat and legible on handwritten forms.
- Date and sign everything. Additionally, be sure to include your credentials along with your signature.
- Follow the procedure dictated by your workplace for correcting errors, both handwritten and electronic.
- Educate yourself on the documentation codes and abbreviations used in your particular workplace.
- Make sure you are competent in basic computer functions like keyboarding and that you are able to successfully navigate the electronic information management system used by your health care facility.
- Maintain your password's confidentiality at all times.
- When using computerized health information systems, always remember to log off when you are no longer using the system.

CHAPTER

4

ETHICS IN HEALTH CARE: THE BASICS

CHAPTER OBJECTIVES | *At the end of this chapter, you should be able to:*

- use and apply ethics-related terminology including morality, ethics, ethical inquiry, ethical principle, ethical challenge, and ethical dilemma
- understand the importance of ethics in the health care workplace
- discuss eight ethical principles in health care
- summarize and analyze health care Code of Ethics documents
- determine appropriate courses of action in ethically challenging health care scenarios

INTRODUCTION

Although the field of ethics is laden with questions and short on conclusive answers, one thing is certain: any time we are dealing with human life, ethical discussion and debate become essential. While health care workers have always dealt with human lives and the complexity of issues that arise as a result, rapid technological developments blur the boundaries of what it means to be human more than ever before and make for some increasingly complex health decisions. In this chapter, you will see that ethical challenges, while "part of the job" for the health care professional, are certainly not an easy part of that job. As you have learned in previous chapters, patient well-being should be the ultimate focus of the health care provider; the achievement of quality patient care can be difficult, however, when other factors compete with and challenge such quality.

In this chapter you will be introduced to terminology that will provide you with the requisite vocabulary to engage in important discussions on the topic of ethics and health. In addition, you will receive an introduction to seven ethical principles commonly used by health care providers to determine appropriate response and behaviour in ethically challenging situations. Finally, you will be asked to apply your understanding of ethics to challenging health care scenarios.

IMPORTANT DEFINITIONS

While **morality** refers to what people believe to be right or wrong, the term **ethics** refers to the analysis and reflection of why we believe something is right or wrong. Consequently, **ethical enquiry** is the process we go through when trying to determine our responses and actions to dilemmas that pose no obvious or easy solutions. An **ethical dilemma** can be defined as a situation where there is conflict between competing **ethical principles**: rules that guide our moral conduct and provide a foundation for ethical decision-making. And, finally, an **ethical challenge** refers to situations where there is a conflict between knowledge and will: situations where one knows the right thing to do but for a variety of reasons, which commonly include fear and/or negative repercussions, is reluctant to act ethically. Ethics, in making us accountable for our moral convictions and our behaviours, allows us to engage in important discussions concerning personal responsibility, professional responsibility, community responsibility, and universal responsibility. Ethics also requires that we consider many important questions when confronted with challenging choices: What is the best course of action in a given situation? Why is this the best course of action? How have I arrived at my decision? What is my decision based on? What should my decision be based on?

ETHICS IN THE HEALTH SCIENCES

In the course of any given day, most workplaces find themselves confronted with ethical challenges or dilemmas and, in the health care workplace, where practitioners deal with matters of mortality and quality of life daily, such scenarios are common. Practising health professionals are constantly placed in situations that require them to examine both their personal and professional consciences in a multitude of areas. What, for example, should a nurse do when asked to participate in a health procedure that he or she morally objects to or disagrees with? What about the massage therapist who is a single parent and struggling financially? How should he respond if asked by a client to perform "extra" services for triple the pay of a therapeutic massage? And then there's the paramedic who is the first on the scene of a violent car crash. How does she handle the lone survivor's request to let him die, after he is told that his wife and child did not survive?

Ethical debate in the field of the health sciences is, of course, not new. Some ethical debates are commonplace and have been discussed and publicized endlessly in schools, colleges, and universities; discussions of whether a fetus should be considered a life or not and the controversies surrounding requests for assisted death or suicide are two such examples. As technology continues to progress, however, health care institutions face increasingly longer, and newer, lists of ethical scenarios to debate and discuss. Modern technology now has the ability to screen developing fetuses for certain birth "defects" and with the option to abort in such circumstances evolves a growing concern over a renewal in eugenicist thinking. With rapid technological growth in the areas of the health sciences, the need to find solutions to new ethical dilemmas posed by these very advancements becomes timely and pressing. Predictably, then, it appears that ethics dialogue will play an increasingly important role in the future of health care institutions. It is a demanding time as health care institutions prepare for a possible re-invention of approaches and attitudes toward life, death, and quality of life. This, along with the limited resources faced by many health care facilities and the increased workloads and greater responsibilities of the practitioners themselves, makes ethics dialogue an increasingly important aspect of health care.

The fact that most college and university health sciences programs require students to take an ethics course, as well as the abundance of textbooks in this area of study, suggests that an understanding of ethics as it relates to health sciences is mandatory for the individual intent on a health sciences career. Ethics dialogue continues beyond the confines of the classroom, however, as, once in the workplace, licensed health professionals in Canada are required to uphold and abide by the Code of Ethics for their particular professions in order to preserve patient rights and dignity.

ETHICAL PRINCIPLES IN HEALTH CARE

As mentioned previously, ethical principles are guidelines that help us navigate the complexities of ethical decision-making by providing a template for model behaviour. The need for ethical guidelines in medical practice has long been recognized as evidenced by creation of the **Hippocratic Oath** (see Box 4.1), a document that set the standards

---

| **BOX 4.1** | **The Hippocratic Oath (Classical Version)** |

I SWEAR by Apollo the physician, and Aesculapius, and Health, and All-heal, and all the gods and goddesses, that, according to my ability and judgment, I will keep this Oath and this stipulation- to reckon him who taught me this Art equally dear to me as my parents, to share my substance with him, and relieve his necessities if required; to look upon his off-spring in the same footing as my own brothers, and to teach them this art, if they shall wish to learn it, without fee or stipulation; and that by precept, lecture, and every other mode of instruction, I will impart a knowledge of the Art to my own sons, and those of my teachers, and to disciples bound by a stipulation and oath according to the law of medicine, but to none others. I will follow that system of regimen which, according to my ability and judgment, I consider for the benefit of my patients, and abstain from whatever is deleterious and mischievous. I will give no deadly medicine to any one if asked, nor suggest any such counsel; and in like manner I will not give to a woman a pessary to produce abortion. With purity and with holiness I will pass my life and practice my Art. I will not cut persons laboring under the stone, but will leave this to be done by men who are practitioners of this work. Into whatever houses I enter, I will go into them for the benefit of the sick, and will abstain from every voluntary act of mischief and corruption; and, further from the seduction of females or males, of freemen and slaves. Whatever, in connection with my professional practice or not, in connection with it, I see or hear, in the life of men, which ought not to be spoken of abroad, I will not divulge, as reckoning that all such should be kept secret. While I continue to keep this Oath unviolated, may it be granted to me to enjoy life and the practice of the art, respected by all men, in all times! But should I trespass and violate this Oath, may the reverse be my lot!

Source: The Oath, by Hippocrates, written 400 B.C.E.; translated by Francis Adams.

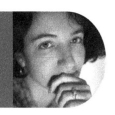

Translation:

Francis Adams

1. Work individually or in groups to rewrite the classical version of the Hippocratic Oath for a modern audience.
2. Does the classical Oath reflect the complexities of the modern health care system? Why or why not?

for ethical medical practice in the fourth century. Today, modernized versions of this ancient document (see Box 4.2) are still used around the world to provide a framework for ethical behaviour. Once you have looked at both versions of the Oath, answer the questions that follow each document.

| BOX 4.2 | The Hippocratic Oath (Modern Version) |

I swear to fulfill, to the best of my ability and judgment, this covenant:
I will respect the hard-won scientific gains of those physicians in whose steps I walk, and gladly share such knowledge as is mine with those who are to follow.
I will apply, for the benefit of the sick, all measures [that] are required, avoiding those twin traps of overtreatment and therapeutic nihilism.

I will remember that there is art to medicine as well as science, and that warmth, sympathy, and understanding may outweigh the surgeon's knife or the chemist's drug.

I will not be ashamed to say "I know not," nor will I fail to call in my colleagues when the skills of another are needed for a patient's recovery.

I will respect the privacy of my patients, for their problems are not disclosed to me that the world may know. Most especially must I tread with care in matters of life and death. If it is given me to save a life, all thanks. But it may also be within my power to take a life; this awesome responsibility must be faced with great humbleness and awareness of my own frailty. Above all, I must not play at God.

I will remember that I do not treat a fever chart, a cancerous growth, but a sick human being, whose illness may affect the person's family and economic stability. My responsibility includes these related problems, if I am to care adequately for the sick.

I will prevent disease whenever I can, for prevention is preferable to cure.

I will remember that I remain a member of society, with special obligations to all my fellow human beings, those sound of mind and body as well as the infirm.

If I do not violate this oath, may I enjoy life and art, respected while I live and remembered with affection thereafter. May I always act so as to preserve the finest traditions of my calling and may I long experience the joy of healing those who seek my help.

Source: Hippocratic Oath, Modern Version. Louis Lasagna, 1964.

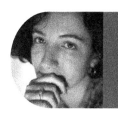

1. Contrast the modern Hippocratic Oath with the classical version. How are the two different?
2. Is there anything in the modern Oath that is missing or that you would like to see included?

Power imbalances lay the foundation for many ethical challenges, and it is virtually impossible to find a profession where hierarchy and power imbalances do not exist to some extent. In health care such power imbalances are obvious when one observes the doctor-nurse relationship or even the nurse-patient relationship. Given such imbalances of power as well as the complexity and frequency of life-determining decisions that health care workers must engage in daily, principles that lay a foundation for helping us determine the best course of action in the face of ethically difficult situations are vital. In the following section, you will be introduced to eight such principles. These principles extend across the health care spectrum and are used, in varying guises, as base guidelines for ethical behaviour in many health professions including nursing, paramedics, physiotherapy, massage therapy, and occupational therapy. These principles, or variations of them, are usually encrypted within a specific profession's Code of Ethics.

1) Autonomy

The principle of autonomy lies at the core of patient rights. Autonomy refers to the right of patients to have a say in all aspects of their personal care: who treats them, how they are treated, and what treatments they choose to undergo or decline. The notion of coercion must also be considered in any discussion of patient autonomy. A caregiver must not attempt to force or coerce a patient into making particular health decisions. Rather, the caregiver must aid in preserving patient autonomy by thoroughly and honestly informing the patient of pertinent matters related to his or her health and treatments so that well-informed health decisions can be made by either the patient or those acting on the patient's behalf. The current emphasis on patient "voice" contrasts with the traditional paternalistic model of health care that assumed expert opinion on the part of the caregiver, oftentimes compromising patient autonomy in the process. The consent form is used by health care institutions to assure autonomy in cases of surgery or other risky treatments. Common categories of consent are explained below.

Implied Consent:

This occurs when a patient consents through words, behaviour, or circumstance. If a patient opens his or her mouth for the purposes of thermometer insertion, this would be considered implied consent through behaviour.

Express Consent:

This refers to written or verbal consent and is usually required when intervention is painful or risky.

Advanced Directives:

An advanced directive falls under the category of express consent and is a written document which expresses how a patient desires to be dealt with in an end of life or crisis situation in the event that he or she is incapable of making his or her own health decisions. Advanced directives may involve specific directions on how to handle an end of life decision or they may simply authorize a specific individual to act on the patient's behalf to make such a decision.

Ethical dilemmas and challenges in the area of autonomy happen frequently in the health care workplace. For example, a patient may assert his or her right to smoke cigarettes despite a serious lung condition. Here, the ethical dilemma for the caregiver becomes one of respecting the patient's right to smoke while at the same time trying to protect the patient from physical harm that might result from his or her right to smoke.

2) Preservation of Life

The underlying tenet inherent in this second principle is that everything possible must be done in order to preserve the well-being and, ultimately, the life of a patient. While this appears to be self-evident, the preservation of life principle can become quite complicated in the realities of the health care workplace in the face of the following questions: What is the definition of life? Should life be defined in purely technical terms, or should it be defined more broadly in terms of quality? If it is determined that an individual can never have quality of life, should that life be preserved? And who determines what quality of life is? Canadian courts know all too well how complex issues relating to the quality of life can get. In the famous 1993 Latimer case, Robert Latimer took the life of his daughter Tracy, determining that she had no quality of life because of her cerebral palsy. Court documents, however, paint a picture of a young girl who smiled and appeared enthusiastic in her interactions with others. Despite these smiles, Robert Latimer determined that his daughter had no quality of life and suffocated and gassed her to death, citing mercy and his daughter's lack of quality of life as his defence (CBC News In Depth, 2008).

Health care workers may, indeed, find themselves confronting situations related to the controversies surrounding definitions of "quality of life." A patient may, for

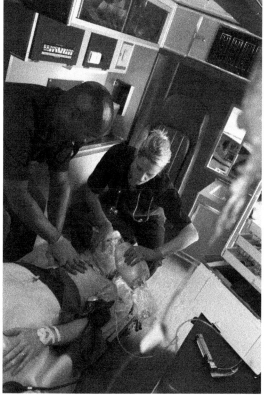

Monkey Business Images/Shutterstock

example, "give up" and resist life-saving procedures, feeling he or she has no quality of life. Such wishes or requests become a dilemma for the health care worker who is supposed to assist in the preservation of life.

3) Beneficence

The principle of beneficence requires caregivers to act beneficently or in ways that benefit their patients and do not produce harm. As well, caregivers must act as advocates for vulnerable patients who cannot "speak" for themselves. In fact, communities come to expect beneficent care from their caregivers and their faith and trust in the medical system centres around this expectation. An ethical dilemma relating to the principle of beneficence might present itself in the case of paramedic dispatch to an attempted suicide. At such a scene, a paramedic may find him- or herself having to perform life-saving procedures on a patient who wants to die. Here, patient autonomy, in this case the patient's desire to die, clashes with the paramedic's obligation to aid and resuscitate the ill.

4) Non-maleficence

In ethical literature, refraining from knowingly harming patients is referred to as non-maleficence. Related to the principle of beneficence, which requires that caregivers protect patients from harm, non-maleficence demands that caregivers should not knowingly cause or inflict harm on their patients. In upholding this principle, caregivers are required to practise and provide information only within the scope of their specialties and not perform or undertake procedures they are not qualified to handle because of potential harm. Health care professionals know all too well, however, that temporarily harming a patient cannot be avoided when medications with side effects or other uncomfortable manifestations have to be administered. The principle of non-maleficence is often challenged in health care. One such scenario includes providing a patient with medication that provides pain relief but which is also known to have addictive properties. In this situation, the health care provider is caught between two ethical principles: acting beneficently toward the patient by working to decrease the patient's pain and not causing future harm to the patient through the administration of an addictive drug.

5) Veracity or Truth Telling

In any relationship, a commitment to honesty is crucial. In the patient–caregiver relationship this is also the case as patient trust forms the cornerstone for patient well-being. If patients do not have trusting relationships with their caregivers, their healing process may be compromised. The potential challenges of veracity become apparent in situations where "the truth hurts." A health care provider might find him- or herself in a situation where revelation of truth would cause great distress to a patient. If, for example, a young mother has just been taken into intensive care after a serious car accident in which her six-month-old infant did not survive, how does a health care team member respond if she questions her child's whereabouts? Should the child's death be disclosed to the mother who is currently experiencing great physical distress? The ethical dilemma arising from this situation involves a conflict between the principles of veracity and beneficence in that caregivers must strive to be truthful toward their patients but also to preserve their patients from harm, both physical and psychological. The principle of veracity extends beyond the confines of the patient–caregiver relationship and includes relationships among the caregivers themselves. Providers must be honest in their dealing with colleagues and managers and must not engage in fraud or cover-up.

6) Confidentiality and Privacy

Many workplaces, like banks and police stations, store sensitive client information. Similarly, the health care provider has access to a variety of sensitive patient information that includes a client's medical and psychological history, all of which must remain confidential. Not revealing the contents of sensitive documents is one thing; retaining privacy in day-to-day interactions with a patient is another. On a day-to-day basis, caregivers are involved intimately with patients in their roles of feeding, bathing, and dressing them. They may witness them crying or screaming as well as see the stresses inherent in their personal relationships during visiting hours. The patient is entitled to privacy throughout all these encounters: curtains should be drawn when performing private procedures and assessments, and the patient's body should always be treated with dignity. In cases where patient health data requires disclosure, written approval is usually necessary. A dilemma that can arise from upholding the principle of confidentiality and privacy is the situation where a patient has, in confidence, revealed life-threatening information to a caregiver. The caregiver now has an ethical dilemma in determining whether to violate the principle of confidentiality in order to preserve the principle of beneficence, if she feels withholding this information could compromise the patient's, or others', health in any way.

7) Justice

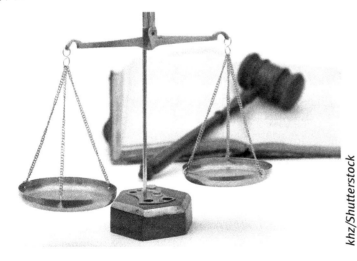

khz/Shutterstock

Justice refers to the principle of fairness that should operate in an ideal society. Justice implies that everyone is entitled to the same level of care and consideration in terms of distribution of resources, access to resources, and so on. The realm of just treatment becomes challenging in a world where health care resources are scarce and the health care provider often has little input in administrative decision-making locally, provincially, and beyond. While Canada's public health care system reflects justice, in theory, with its emphasis on universality and accessibility, inequities still occur, with some people being unable to afford expenses not covered by provincial health plans. Justice as it relates to health care can be divided into two types:

Distributive justice:

This type of justice demands that resources and taxation be distributed fairly and properly. It also demands equality of treatment in terms of sex, race, economic class, and the like.

Compensatory justice:

This type of justice refers to the recognition of harm and the responsibility of just societies to compensate individuals for wrongdoing.

A challenge that might arise relating to the principle of justice includes the knowledge of unequal treatment. Perhaps a nurse has noticed that the doctor for whom she works treats his white patients better than his oriental patients. The nurse finds herself in an ethical challenge as she is required by her profession to uphold the principle of justice which calls for the equal treatment of all, but at the same time she is reluctant to get into "hot water" with her superior who has more professional power than she does and with whom she must work on a daily basis.

8) Fidelity

The principle of fidelity demands behaviour that demonstrates loyalty and faithfulness toward patients. As such, this principle summarizes many of the expectations inherent in several of the other principles already mentioned. Above all, this principle requires caregivers to uphold with integrity the responsibilities that result from their designations as licensed health care providers. This principle also includes the expectation that contracts be respected and honoured. If a patient agrees to a procedure, the doers of that procedure have the obligation to conduct that procedure professionally and properly. Challenges in the area of fidelity are numerous in the health care workplace. One example would be the nurse who is required to assist in an abortion procedure when she herself does not believe in abortion. In this situation, the nurse's fidelity to her profession is challenged by her personal beliefs.

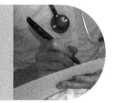

It's always difficult when family members want you to keep resuscitating a patient even when you know such efforts are fruitless. I've had to do all sorts of crazy things, and I mean crazy, just to appease family members who are

not ready to let their loved ones go. Sometimes, because family members are not ready to deal with loss, they want us to keep putting the patient through excruciating pain and discomfort. This seems selfish to me. Love also means "letting go."

—RPN, (hospital)

TRY IT YOURSELF

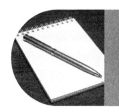

What ethical principle is being questioned or asserted in each of the following scenarios? Some scenarios might reflect more than one principle.

1. A patient no longer wants to live and asks that he no longer be resuscitated.

2. A massage therapist who has a family wedding to go to on the weekend has been asked by her manager to work overtime on the same weekend.

3. A paramedic team having coffee at Tim Hortons openly discusses the health of a local celebrity they just transported to the hospital.

4. A patient wants a second opinion on her health diagnosis.

5. A nurse offers to sit with a patient on his lunch break because he sees that the patient is distressed.

6. A patient does not come for his regular medical checkups because he cannot afford the transit to get to the hospital.

7. A nurse speaks to her manager about concerns she has regarding lack of staffing in her ward.

8. A nurse knows that the husband of one of her patients is having an affair with another nurse on the ward.

9. A patient rejects a life-saving blood transfusion on religious grounds.

10. A patient is distressed about an upcoming surgery. The nurse tells the patient that "Dr. Harris is the best. You'll come out of the surgery feeling like you're twenty years old".

THE CODE OF ETHICS DOCUMENT

Now that you have been introduced to common ethical principles in health care, it is time to look at some actual Code of Ethics documents found in the health care workplace. It is important to note that even if a health workplace does not have an official Code of Ethics document, workers must still act ethically and honourably in order to uphold the standards of their professions as well as the dignity of their patients. Below you will find actual Code of Ethics documents for three professions: nursing (Box 4.3), paramedics (Box 4.4), and physiotherapy (Box 4.5). As you read each profession's code, see how many ethical principles discussed in this chapter you can find.

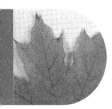

BOX 4.3 Code of Ethics for Registered Nurses

1. ... Providing safe, compassionate, competent and ethical care
2. Promoting health and well-being
3. Promoting and respecting informed decision-making
4. Preserving dignity
5. Maintaining privacy and confidentiality
6. Promoting justice
7. Being accountable ...

Source: © 2008, Canadian Nurses Association. May not be reproduced without written permission of the copyright owner.

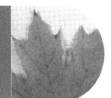

BOX 4.4 Code of Ethics for Paramedics (Manitoba)

The Paramedic Association of Manitoba affirms its responsibility to develop the spirit of professionalism within its membership and to promote high ethical standards in the practice of Emergency Medical Services.

Paramedic Association of Manitoba members are committed to achieving excellence:

I. The paramedic shall regard their responsibility to the patient as paramount and strive to preserve human life, alleviate suffering, and adhere to the principles of beneficence. The paramedic must have respect for their patients' autonomy and ensure quality and equal availability of care to all.

II. The paramedic shall provide services based on human need, with respect for human dignity, unrestricted by consideration of age, race, sex, color, status, national or ethnic origin, or physical/mental disability.

III. The paramedic shall respect, protect, and fulfill the commitment to confidentiality of patient information in accordance with law.

IV. The paramedic shall practice their profession uninfluenced by motives of profit.

V. The paramedic will assume all responsibility for his or her actions, and ensure that others receive credit for their work and contributions.

VI. The paramedic assumes responsibility to expose incompetence or unethical conduct of others to the appropriate authority. The paramedic refuses to participate in unethical procedures.

VII. Each practitioner understands and complies with the laws and regulations relevant to their professional role.

VIII. The paramedic shall participate in defining and upholding standards of professional practice and education. The paramedic strives for professional excellence by maintaining competence in knowledge and skills necessary to provide quality care and maintaining currency in issues related to EMS.

IX. The paramedic recognizes a responsibility to participate in professional activities, associations, and research that contribute to the improvement of public health, and will and encourage the participation of peers.

This code of ethics is not law, but a professional standard of conduct which defines the essentials of honorable behaviour for the paramedic; a behaviour that will foster pride, admiration, and respect for the profession of paramedicine.

Source: Courtesy of the Paramedic Association of Manitoba

BOX 4.5   Code of Ethics for Physiotherapists

Premise:

The provision of effective quality care, while respecting the rights of the client, shall be the primary consideration of each member of the profession.

Responsibilities to the Client

1. Physiotherapists shall respect the client's rights, dignity, needs, wishes and values.
2. Physiotherapists may not refuse care to any client on grounds of race, religion, ethnic or national origin, age, sex, sexual orientation, and social or health status.
3. Physiotherapists must respect the client's or surrogate's right to be informed about the effects of treatment and inherent risks.
4. Physiotherapists must give clients or surrogates the opportunity to consent to or decline treatment or alterations in the treatment regime.
5. Physiotherapists shall confine themselves to clinical diagnosis and management in those aspects of physiotherapy in which they have been educated and which are recognized by the profession. (Physiotherapists are responsible for recognizing and practising within their levels of competence. The clinical diagnosis is established by taking a history and conducting a physical and functional examination. The identification of the client's problems and the physiotherapeutic management is based on this diagnosis in conjunction with an understanding of pertinent biopsychosocial factors. This rule does not restrict the expansion of the scope of physiotherapy practice.)
6. Physiotherapists shall assume full responsibility for all care they provide.

7. Physiotherapists shall not treat clients when the medical diagnosis or clinical condition indicates that the commencement or continuation of physiotherapy is not warranted or is contraindicated.

8. Physiotherapists shall request consultation with, or refer clients to, colleagues or members of other health professions when, in the opinion of the physiotherapist, such action is in the best interest of the client.

9. Physiotherapists shall document the client's history and relevant subjective information, the physiotherapist's objective findings, clinical diagnosis, treatment plan and procedures, explanation to the client, progress notes and discharge summary.

10. Physiotherapists shall respect all client information as confidential. Such information shall not be communicated to any person without the consent of the client or surrogate except when required by law.

11. Physiotherapists, with the client's or surrogate's consent, may delegate specific aspects of the care of that client to a person deemed by the physiotherapist to be competent to carry out the care safely and effectively.

12. Physiotherapists are responsible for all duties they delegate to personnel under their supervision.

Source: Canadian Physiotherapy Association, Responsibilities to the client: Rules of Conduct, 1988.

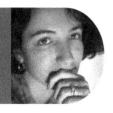

PRACTICE: ETHICAL DISCUSSIONS

You have now had a chance to review and analyze several Code of Ethics documents. Based on your knowledge of the various codes, work individually, in pairs, or in groups to discuss appropriate responses to each of the scenarios below. Be prepared to justify your responses and decisions using the relevant Code of Ethics.

Case 1: The Negligent Colleague

Rosalind Gonzales and Hema Bannerjee are both experienced registered nurses. They have been working together in the same hospital for 15 years. In addition to being long-time colleagues, Gonzales and Bannerjee are also good friends. They socialize frequently, and three years ago Gonzales lent Bannerjee a significant sum of money for an important car repair.

Recently, Bannerjee has become concerned about Gonzales' professional conduct. Gonzales, a normally professional, competent, and popular nurse with the patients, has started to look tired and arrives late to work. Bannerjee noticed Gonzales tripping while wheeling a patient down the hall the other day, and today she is sure that she smelled alcohol on her colleague's breath in the lunch cafeteria. She has also noticed that Gonzales has been negligent in some of her charting duties. In fact, Bannerjee herself has had to approach Gonzales on more than one occasion this week concerning some vague and confusing notations made on a shared patient's chart. Bannerjee is starting to worry that her friend and colleague may be an alcoholic.

Discussion Questions:

1. What ethical principle or principles are at play here?

2. What specific ethical challenge or challenges does Bannerjee face?

3. What would you do in this situation? Justify your response.

4. Based on the Code of Ethics for nurses, what should Bannerjee do in this situation? Justify your response.

Case 2: The Abusive Patient

Saba Hassan is a physiotherapist who was just recently hired at a popular community health clinic. Because she is a new employee at the clinic, she is under intense scrutiny and must serve a one-year probation period. Hassan loves her job and looks forward to seeing her patients and monitoring their progress. For the past week, however, she has felt anxious in having to deal with one particular patient: Horatio Littleton. Littleton, who is healing from a broken leg, comes for therapy three times a week. So far, Littleton has made several sexual comments about Hassan's body and has tried to grope her while she was helping him with his leg exercises. Hassan finds his inappropriate behaviour highly distressing. Hassan has noticed that she is short and abrasive when interacting with Littleton as well as shaking with anxiety prior to treating him.

Discussion Questions:

1. What ethical principle or principles are at play here?

2. What specific ethical challenge or challenges does Hassan face?

3. What would you do in this situation? Justify your response.

4. Based on the Code of Ethics for physiotherapists, what should Hassan do? Justify your response.

Case 3: The Grateful Patient

Paramedic Lucien Godbout and his ambulance partner James Pauley have just arrived at the apartment building of an elderly gentleman who called 911 complaining of a fall and a broken hip. Upon arrival, Godbout and Pauley examine the patient and conclude the patient's self-assessment is correct: he has a broken hip. The two paramedics strap the patient onto a stretcher in order to transport him to the ambulance downstairs. As they are exiting the apartment, the patient thrusts a $100 bill into Godbout's hands. "You remind me so much of my son," he says. "Here, take this, I might not see you again. You have been so nice."

Discussion Questions:

1. What ethical principle or principles are at play here?

2. What specific ethical challenge or challenges does Godbout face?

3. What would you do in this situation? Justify your response.

4. Based on the Code of Ethics for paramedics, what should Godbout do? Justify your response.

Case 4: The Abused Patient

Tatiana Gruszinksy is a registered nurse working in the ER department of her local hospital. Gruszinksy is on duty one night when she sees her best friend and her 10-year-old daughter in the waiting room. Gruszinksy ends up being responsible for assessing her friend's daughter before the doctor's arrival. During her examination, she discovers several bruises on the child's body; her extensive professional experience tells her these bruises are the results of physical abuse. Gruszinksy is very distressed by these findings. Her best friend, the child's mother, is attempting to make small talk while the examination is taking place.

Discussion Questions:

1. What ethical principle or principles are at play here?

2. What specific ethical challenge or challenges does Gruszinksy face?

3. What would you do in this situation? Justify your response.

4. Based on the Code of Ethics for nurses, what should Gruszinksy do? Justify your response.

Case 5: The Unlikeable Patient

Lance Fisher is a paramedic who was just dispatched to the scene of a violent home invasion. Upon arrival, he discovers a female who has been raped as well as her rapist, who is lying in a pool of blood with a stab wound to his stomach. Despite paramedic and police presence, the rapist continues to yell obscenities at his victim. Fisher, who has a wife and two teenage daughters, is disgusted at the thought of having to save this rapist's life.

Discussion Questions:

1. What ethical principle or principles are at play here?

2. What specific ethical challenge or challenges does Fisher face?

3. What would you do in this situation? Justify your response.

4. Based on the Code of Ethics for paramedics, what should Fisher do? Justify your response.

CHAPTER 5

CREATIVE CONNECTIONS: HEALTH DISCUSSIONS AND CONTROVERSIES

At the end of this chapter, you should be able to:

- critically think about issues related to illness, aging, disability, death, and disease
- express your opinions on a variety of health issues thoughtfully, confidently, and diplomatically
- engage in meaningful discussions related to health and health care
- recognize the importance of the reflective process in health care and how analysis and discussion of fiction can enhance that process
- format APA reference citations correctly by following model samples

INTRODUCTION

The information in the previous four chapters focused mainly on helping you meet the technical requirements of your health science certificate or degree as well as equipped you for the formalities of the workplace. To be successful, a health care worker requires more than technical knowledge, however. In working with individuals in very vulnerable situations, you must also be prepared to exercise traits of patience, tolerance, compassion, understanding, and empathy. In this last chapter, you will explore and reflect upon your capacity for these traits in a unique, interesting, and thought-provoking way: through the analysis of poetry, short stories, and film.

The arts have a mesmerizing power. A story, poem, or film often seduces us because we empathize and can relate to its contents in meaningful ways. Art is about our lives and, as such, it proves the perfect medium through which to reflect on health-related themes like aging, disability, illness, disease, and death. Reflecting on such issues is an important process for the health care provider who finds him- or herself in the centre of an emotionally charged environment filled with grief, apathy, conflict, and pain. And, as a professional, you must navigate this complex emotional world with success, dignity, and grace. By reading and thinking about the story, poetry, and film selections that follow, you will, hopefully, gain deeper insight and understanding into the complexities of the human condition, a necessary and important step for anyone interested in the health care field.

Even though the majority of characters you will encounter in this chapter are fictitious, their struggles in the areas of illness, isolation, aging, relationships, and health care reflect real-world conflicts and concerns. As you explore the stories, poems, and films herein, you will have much to contemplate long after you leave the classroom.

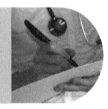

I remember reading a story by Vincent Lam called "Night Flight" in one of my communication classes when I was studying to be a paramedic. It was about a helicopter medic who was off to save a dying man in Guatemala. The story was amazing; it seemed so real. As I read the story, I really felt the stresses and the fast pace of the medic's lifestyle. Once I read that story, I knew that I was in the right field. I've even gone on to read other books by Lam, and they continue to give me insights into my work, now that I'm a practising paramedic. Stories educate and inspire me in a way that boring textbooks just can't.

—Paramedic graduate, Humber College

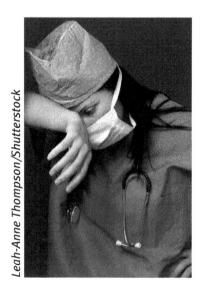

Leah-Anne Thompson/Shutterstock

STORIES TO ANALYZE AND DISCUSS

The following two stories, Doris Lessing's "Casualty" (1992) and Linda Svendsen's "White Shoulders" (1992), provide useful and provocative insights into the world of illness and health care. With the incorporation of diverse themes like illness, suicide, grief, and nursing, both stories are rich in material to discuss and debate. In "Casualty", Lessing's fictitious emergency waiting room provides a relevant and useful critique of the real-world hospital, highlighting the frustrations of both patients and staff in the process. In "White Shoulders" a family member's diagnosis of cancer wreaks further devastation on an already dysfunctional family. Read each story carefully and then work in small groups to discuss the questions that follow each reading.

"CASUALTY" by Doris Lessing

All of them looking one way, they sat on metal chairs, the kind that are hard and slippery and stack into each other. They kept their attention on the woman behind the reception desk, who was apparently not interested in them now she had their names, addresses, complaints all tidily written down on forms. She was an ample young woman with the rainy violet eyes that seem designed only for laughing or weeping, but now they were full of the stern impartiality of justice. Her name button said she was Nurse Doolan.

It was a large room with walls an uninteresting shade of beige, bare except for the notice, "If You Have Nothing Urgently Wrong Please Go To Your Own Doctor." Evidently the twenty or so people here did not believe their own doctors were as good as this hospital casualty department. Only one of them seemed in urgent need, a dishevelled woman of forty or so with dyed orange hair, who was propping her wrapped left hand on her right shoulder. Everyone knew the wrist was broken because the woman with her had nodded commandingly at them, turning round to do it, and mouthed, "Her wrist. She broke it." Satisfied they must all acknowledge precedence, she had placed her charge in the end of the front row nearest to the door that said "No Admittance." They did not challenge her. The broken-wristed one, exhausted with pain, drowsed in her seat, and her face was bluish white, so that with the brush of orange hair she looked like a clown. But Nurse Doolan did not seem to think she deserved more than the others, for when the next name was called it was not the owner of the wrist. "Harkness," said Nurse Doolan and while an apparently fit young man walked into "No Admittance" the poor clown's attendant stood up and complained, "But it is urgent, it is a broken wrist."

"Won't be long," said Nurse Doolan, and placidly studied her pile of forms.

"They don't care. They don't care at all," said an old woman in a wheelchair. Her voice was loud and accusing. She was fat and looked like a constipated frog. Her face, full of healthy colour, showed a practised resignation to life's taunts. "I fell down a good six hours ago, and my shoulder's broke, I know that!" The elderly woman sitting with her did not try to engage anyone's sympathy, but rather avoided eyes that had already clearly said, Rather you than me! She said quietly, "It's all right, Auntie, don't go on."

"Don't go on, she says," said the old woman, eighty if she was a day, and full of energy. "It's all right for some."

A boy of about twelve emerged from the mysteries behind "No Admittance" with a crutch and a bandaged foot, and was guided through this waiting room to the outside pavement by a nurse who left him there, presumably to be picked up. She came back.

"Nurse," said the old woman, "my shoulder's broke and I've been sitting here for hours . . . ever so long," she added, as her relative murmured, "Not long, Auntie, only half an hour."

This nurse glanced towards Doolan at Reception, who signalled with her violet eyes. Nurse Bates, directed, stopped by the wheelchair and switched on appropriate sympathy. "Let's have a look," she said.

The elderly niece drew back part of a bright pink cardigan from the shoulder which sat there, stoutly and soberly bare, except for a grimy shoulder strap. "You want me naked, I suppose that's it now! For everyone to gape at! That's it, I suppose!" The nurse bent over the shoulder, gently manipulating it, while everybody stared somewhere else, so as not to give the old horror the satisfaction of feeling looked at.

"Owwwww," wailed the old woman.

"You'll live," said the nurse briskly, straightening herself.

"It's broken, isn't it?" urged Auntie.

"You've got a bit of a bruise, but that's about it, I think. They'll find out in X-ray." And she stepped smartly off towards "No Admittance," raising her brows and smiling with her eyes at Nurse Doolan, who smiled with hers.

"They don't care," came the loud voice. "None of them care. How'd you like to be lying on the floor by yourself half the night and no one near you to lift you up?"

The elderly niece, a thin and colourless creature who probably— though for her sake everyone hoped not—devoted her life to this old bully, did not bother to defend herself, but smoothed back the pink cardigan over the shoulder which if you looked hard did have a mauveish shine.

"Day after day, sitting by myself, I might as well be dead."

"Would you like a cup of tea, Auntie?"

"Might as well, if you'll put yourself out. Not that it'll be worth drinking."

The niece allowed her face to show a moment's exhaustion as she turned away from Auntie, but then she smiled and went through the rows of waiting people with "Excuse me, excuse me, please."

"Fanshawe," said Nurse Doolan, apparently in reply to some summons in the ether, for no one had come out.

A man of sixty-five or so, who wore a red leather slipper on one foot, used a stick to heave himself up, and walked slowly to the inner door, careful the stick did not slip.

"You'd think they'd have nonslip floors," came from the wheelchair.

"They are nonslip," said Doolan firmly.

"Better be safe than sorry," said Mr. Fanshawe, going into "No Admittance" with a wink all round that meant he wasn't going to be associated with that old bitch.

"And what about my sister?" asked the woman who was now cradling the broken-wristed one. Her voice trembled, and she seemed about to weep with indignation.

And indeed the poor clown seemed half conscious, her orange head drooping, then jerking up, then falling forward, and she even groaned. She heard herself groan and embarrassment woke her up. She flashed painful smiles along the front row, and as far as she could turn her head to the back. "I fell," she muttered, confessing it, begging forgiveness. "I fell, you see."

"You're not the only one to fall," came from the wheelchair.

"There's been a bad accident," said Nurse Doolan. "They've been working in there like navvies these last three hours."

"Oh, that's it, is it?" "That's what it is, then!" "Oh well, in that case..." came from the longsuffering crowd.

"Never seen anything like it," said Nurse Doolan, sharing this with them.

It was noticeable that she and some others glanced nervously at the old woman, who decided not to have her say, not this time. And here was her niece with her tea in the plastic foam cup.

"And what did I tell you?" demanded Auntie, taking the cup and at once noisily gulping the tea. "Plastic rubbish and it's cold, you'd think. . . ."

A trundling sound from inside "No Admittance." As the doors opened there emerged the back of a young black porter in his natty uniform, then a steel trolley, and on the trolley a human form rolled in bandages to the waist, but naked above and showing a strong healthy young man's chest. Black. From the neck began a cocoon: a white bandaged head. Alert brown eyes looked out from the cocoon. The trolley disappeared into the interior of the hospital on its way to some ward several floors up.

"The wrist," said Nurse Doolan, "Bisley," and the woman with the broken wrist was urged to her feet by her sister, and stood swaying. Doolan at once pressed a bell which they heard shrilling inside "No Admittance." The same nurse came running out, saw why she had been summoned, and with Nurse Bates on one side and her sister on the other the half-conscious Wrist was supported within.

Now a new addition to the morning's casualties. In came two young women, made up and dressed up as if off to a disco, chattering away and apparently in the best of health. They lowered their voices, sensing that their jollity was not being appreciated, and sat at the very back, whispering and sometimes giggling. What could they be doing in Casualty?

It seemed that at any moment this was what the old woman would start asking, for she was fixing them with a hard, cold, accusing look. "Auntie," said her niece hastily, "would you like another tea? I could do with one myself."

"I don't mind." And she graciously handed over her cup. The niece went out again.

And then, everything changed. A group of young men appeared outside the glass doors to the world where cars came and went, where visitors walked past, where there was ordinariness and health. This group sent waves of urgency and alarm into the waiting room even before the doors opened.

A young workman in white overalls blotched with red stood gripping the edge of a door because over his shoulder lay a body, and it was heavy, as they could all see, being limp and with no fight in it. This body was a young man too, but his white overalls were soaked with a dreadful dark pulsing blood that still welled from somewhere.

"Why didn't you..." began Nurse Doolan, on her way to saying, "You're not supposed to come in at that door, you need a stretcher, this isn't at all how we do things..." Something on these lines, but no one would ever know, for having taken one look at what was before them, she put her thumb down on the bell to make it shrill in the ears of the doctors and nurses working inside out of sight.

Feet and voices, and out came running the same nurse; three doctors—two women and a man—and a porter with a stretcher.

Seeing the group of young men just inside the door these professionals all stopped still, and the main woman doctor waved aside the stretcher.

"He fell off the roof," said the young man who held his mate. "He fell off." He sounded incredulous, appealing to them, the experts, to say that this was impossible and could not have happened. His mate at his elbow, a youth whose sky-blue overalls had no spot or stain, corroborated, "Yes, he fell off. Suddenly he wasn't there. And then..." Another youth, following behind, still held a paint roller in one hand. Orange paint. These three young men were about twenty, certainly not more than twenty-two or twenty-three. They were pale, shocked, and their eyes told everyone they had seen something terrible and could not stop looking at it.

The woman doctor in charge summoned the group forward, and the doctors and nurse stood to one side as the young men went through into "No Admittance." Blood pattered down.

And then they were all able to see the face that hung over the blood-soaked shoulder. It was dull grey, not a colour many of them were likely to have seen on a face. The mouth hung open. The eyes were open. Blue eyes... The professionals followed the young men in, and the doors swung shut.

Nurse Doolan came out from behind the desk with a cloth, and bent to wipe blood off the floor. She too looked sick.

Meanwhile the second cup of tea arrived, and the old woman took it. The niece, feeling that something had happened in the few minutes she had been gone, was looking around, but no one looked at her. They stared at "No Admittance," and their faces were full of news.

"Well," said the old woman loudly, full of gleeful energy. "I haven't done badly at that, have I? I am eighty-five this year and there's plenty more where that came from!"

No one looked at her, and no one said anything.

Source: "Casualty" from The Real Thing. © 1992 Doris Lessing. Reprinted by kind permission of Jonathan Clowes Lts., London, on behalf of Doris Lessing.

Model APA Citation:

Lessing, D. (1997). Casualty. In B. Meyer (Ed.), *The stories: Contemporary short fiction written in English* (pp. 353–357). Scarborough, ON: Prentice Hall. (Original work published 1987)

Discussion Questions:

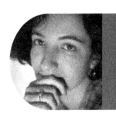

1. What does the title "Casualty" refer to?

2. The author appears to be criticizing the hospital emergency waiting room. What exactly are her criticisms?

3. Based on your personal experiences in the Canadian hospital, do you think Lessing's portrayal of the emergency waiting room is realistic and accurate? Why or why not?

4. What do the patients complain about? Why?

5. How do the nurses treat and respond to the patients? Why?

6. Does the author's bias come through in the story? That is, do you think the author sympathizes more with the patients or the nurses? Why?

7. What is meant by "appropriate sympathy"?

8. Why is the phrase "No Admittance" repeated in the story?

9. At one point in the story the author writes, "And then, everything changed". What exactly changes at this point in the story?

10. What do you think Lessing wants us to understand about the world of health care from "Casualty"?

"WHITE SHOULDERS" by Linda Svendsen

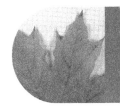

My oldest sister's name is Irene de Haan and she has never hurt anybody. She lives with cancer, in remission, and she has stayed married to the same undemonstrative Belgian Canadian, a brake specialist, going on thirty years. In the family's crumbling domestic empire, Irene and Peter's union has been, quietly, and despite tragedy, what our mother calls the lone success.

Back in the late summer of 1984, before Irene was admitted into hospital for removal of her left breast, I flew home from New York to Vancouver to be with her. We hadn't seen each other for four years, and since I didn't start teaching ESL night classes until mid-September, I was free, at loose ends, unlike the rest of her family. Over the past months, Peter had used up vacation and personal days shuttling her to numerous tests, but finally had to get back to work. He still had a mortgage. Their only child, Jill, who'd just turned seventeen, was entering her last year of high school. Until junior high, she'd been one of those unnaturally well-rounded kids—taking classes in the high dive, water ballet, drawing, and drama, and boy-hunting in the mall on Saturdays with a posse of dizzy friends. Then, Irene said, overnight she became unathletic, withdrawn, and bookish: an academic drone. At any rate, for Jill and Pete's sake, Irene didn't intend to allow her illness to interfere with their life. She wanted everything to proceed as normally as possible. As who wouldn't.

In a way, and this will sound callous, the timing had worked out. Earlier that summer, my ex-husband had been offered a temporary teaching position across the country, and after a long dinner at our old Szechuan dive, I'd agreed to temporarily revise our custody arrangement. With his newfound bounty, Bill would rent a California town house for nine months and royally support the kids. 'Dine and Disney,' he'd said.

I'd blessed this, but then missed them. I found myself dead asleep in the middle of the day in Jane's lower bunk, or tuning in late afternoon to my six-year-old son's, and Bill's, obsession, *People's Court*. My arms ached when I saw other women holding sticky hands, pulling frenzied children along behind them in the August dog days. So I flew west. To be a mother again, I'd jokingly told Irene over the phone. To serve that very need.

Peter was late meeting me at the airport. We gave each other a minimal hug, and then he shouldered my bags and walked ahead out into the rain. The Datsun was double-parked, hazards flashing, with a homemade sign taped on the rear window that said STUD. DRIVER. 'Jill,' he said, loading the trunk. 'Irene's been teaching her so she can pick up the groceries. Help out for a change.' I got in, he turned on easy-listening, and we headed north towards the grey mountains.

Irene had been in love with him since I was a child; he'd been orphaned in Belgium during World War II, which moved both Irene and our mother. He'd also reminded us of Emile, the Frenchman in *South Pacific*, because he was greying, autocratic, and seemed misunderstood. But the European charm had gradually worn thin; over the years, I'd been startled by Peter's racism and petty tyranny. I'd often wished that the young Irene had been fondled off her two feet by a breadwinner more tender, more local. Nobody else in the family agreed and Mum even hinted that I'd become bitter since the demise of my own marriage.

'So how is she?' I finally asked Peter.

'She's got a cold,' he said, 'worrying herself sick. And other than that, it's hard to say.' His tone was markedly guarded. He said prospects were poor; the lump was large and she had the fast-growing, speedy sort of cancer. 'But she thinks the Paki quack will get it when he cuts,' he said.

I sat with that. 'And how's Jill?'

'Grouchy,' he said. 'Bitchy.' This gave me pause, and it seemed to have the same effect on him.

We pulled into the garage of the brick house they'd lived in since Jill's birth, and he waved me on while he handled the luggage. The house seemed smaller now, tucked under tall Douglas firs and fringed with baskets of acutely pink geraniums and baby's breath. The back door was open, so I walked in; the master bedroom door was ajar, but I knocked first. She wasn't there. Jill called, 'Aunt Adele?' and I headed back down the hall to the guestroom, and stuck my head in.

A wan version of my sister rested on a water bed in the dark. When I plunked down I made a tiny wave. Irene almost smiled. She was thin as a fine chain; in my embrace, her flesh barely did the favour of keeping her bones company. Her blondish hair was quite short, and she looked ordinary, like a middle-aged matron who probably worked at a bank and kept a no-fail punch recipe filed away. I had to hold her, barely, close again. Behind us, the closet was full of her conservative garments—flannel, floral—and I understood that this was her room now. She slept here alone. She didn't frolic with Peter any more, have sex.

'Don't cling,' Irene said slowly, but with her old warmth. 'Don't get melodramatic. I'm not dying. It's just a cold.'

'Aunt Adele,' Jill said.

I turned around; I'd forgotten my niece was even there, and she was sitting right on the bed, wedged against a bolster. We kissed hello with loud smooch effects—our ritual—and while she kept a hand on Irene's shoulder, she stuttered answers to my questions about school and her summer. Irene kept an eye on a mute TV—the U.S. Open—although she didn't have much interest in tennis; I sensed, really, that she didn't have any extra energy available for banter. This was conservation, not rudeness.

Jill looked different. In fact, the change in her appearance and demeanour exceeded the ordinary drama of puberty; she seemed to be another girl—sly, unsure, and unable to look in the eye. She wore silver wire glasses, no makeup, jeans with an oversize kelly-green sweatshirt, and many extra pounds. Her soft strawcoloured hair was pulled back with a swan barrette, the swan's eye downcast. When she passed Irene a glass of water and a pill, Irene managed to swallow, then passed it back, and Jill drank, too. To me, it seemed she took great care, twisting the glass in her hand, to sip from the very spot her mother's lips had touched.

Peter came in, sat down on Jill's side of the bed, and stretched both arms around to raise the back of his shirt. He bared red, hairless skin, and said, 'Scratch.'

'But I'm watching tennis,' Jill said softly.

'But you're my daughter,' he said. 'And I have an itch.'

Peter looked at Irene and she gave Jill a sharp nudge. 'Do your poor dad,' she said. 'You don't even have to get up.'

'But aren't I watching something?' Jill said. She glanced around, searching for an ally.

'*Vrouw*,' Peter spoke up. 'This girl, she doesn't do anything except mope, eat, mope, eat.'

Jill's shoulders sagged slightly, as if all air had suddenly abandoned her body, and then she slowly got up. 'I'll see you after, Aunt Adele,' she whispered, and I said, 'Yes, sure,' and then she walked out.

Irene looked dismally at Peter; he made a perverse sort of face—skewing his lips south. Then she reached over and started to scratch his bare back. It was an effort. 'Be patient with her, Peter,' she said. 'She's worried about the surgery.'

'She's worried you won't be around to wait on her,' Peter said, then instructed, 'Go a little higher.' Irene's fingers crept obediently up. 'Tell Adele what Jill said.'

Irene shook her head. 'I don't remember.'

Peter turned to me. 'When Irene told her about the cancer, she said, "Don't die on me, Mum, or I'll kill you." And she said this so serious. Can you imagine?' Peter laughed uninhibitedly, and then Irene joined in, too, although her quiet accompaniment was forced. There wasn't any recollected pleasure in her eyes at all; rather, it seemed as if she didn't want Peter to laugh alone, to appear as odd as he did. 'Don't die or I'll kill you,' Peter said.

* * *

Irene had always been private about her marriage. If there were disagreements with Peter, and there had been—I'd once dropped in unannounced and witnessed a string of Christmas lights whip against the fireplace and shatter—they were never rebroadcast to the rest of the family; if she was ever discouraged or lonely, she didn't confide in anyone, unless she kept a journal or spoke to her God. She had never said a word against the man.

The night before Irene's surgery, after many earnest wishes and ugly flowers had been delivered, she asked me to stay late with her at Lion's Gate Hospital. The room had emptied. Peter had absconded with Jill—and she'd gone reluctantly, asking to stay until I left—and our mother, who'd been so nervous and sad that an intern had fed her Valium from his pocket, 'why is this happening to her?' Mum said to him. 'To my only happy child.'

Irene, leashed to an IV, raised herself to the edge of the bed and looked out at the parking lot and that kind Pacific twilight. 'That Jill,' Irene said. She allowed her head to fall, arms crossed in front of her. 'She should lift a finger for her father.'

'Well,' I said, watching my step, aware she needed peace, 'Peter's not exactly the most easygoing.'

'No,' she said weakly.

We sat for a long time, Irene in her white gown, me beside her in my orange-and-avocado track suit, until I began to think I'd been too tough on Peter and had distressed her. Then she spoke. 'Sometimes I wish I'd learned more Dutch,' she said neutrally. 'When I met Peter, we married not speaking the same language, really. And that made a difference.'

She didn't expect a comment—she raised her head and stared out the half-open window—but I was too shocked to respond anyway. I'd never heard her remotely suggest that her and Peter's marriage had been less than a living storybook. 'You don't like him, do you?' she said. 'You don't care for his Belgian manner.'

I didn't answer; it didn't need to be said aloud. I turned away. 'I'm probably not the woman who can best judge these things,' I said.

Out in the hall, a female patient talked on the phone. Irene and I both listened. 'I left it in the top drawer,' she said wearily. 'No. The *bedroom*.' There was a pause. 'The desk in the hall, try that.' Another pause. 'Then ask Susan where she put it, because I'm tired of this and I need it.' I turned as she hung the phone up and saw her check to see if money had tumbled back. The hospital was quiet again. Irene did not move, but she was shaking; I found it difficult to watch this and reached out and took her hand.

'What is it?' I said. 'Irene.'

She told me she was scared. Not for herself, but for Peter. That when she had first explained to him about the cancer, he hadn't spoken to her for three weeks. Or touched her. Or kissed her. He'd slept in the guestroom, until she'd offered to move there. And he'd been after Jill to butter his toast, change the sheets, iron his pants. Irene had speculated about this, she said, until she'd realized he was acting this way because of what had happened to him when he was little. In Belgium. Bruges, the war. He had only confided in her once. He'd said all the women he'd ever loved had left him. His mother killed, his sister. 'And now me,' Irene said. 'The big C which leads to the big D. If I move on, I leave two children. And I've told Jill they have to stick together.'

I got off the bed. 'But Irene,' I said, 'she's not on earth to please her father. Who can be unreasonable. In my opinion.'

By this time, a medical team was touring the room. The junior member paused by Irene and said, 'Give me your vein.'

'In a minute,' she said to him, 'please,' and he left. There were dark areas, the colour of new bruises, under her eyes. 'I want you to promise me something.'

'Yes.'

'If I die,' she said, 'and I'm not going to, but if I do, I don't want Jill to live with you in New York. Because that's what she wants to do. I want her to stay with Peter. Even if she runs to you, send her back.'

'I can't promise that,' I said. 'Because you're not going to go anywhere.'

She looked at me. Pale, fragile. She was my oldest sister, who'd always been zealous about the silver lining in that cloud; and now it seemed she might be dying, in her forties—too soon—and she needed to believe I could relieve her of this burden. So I nodded, *Yes*.

* * *

When I got back, by cab, to Irene and Peter's that night, the house was dark. I groped up the back steps, ascending through a hovering scent of honeysuckle, stepped inside, and turned on the kitchen light. The TV was going—some ultra-loud camera commercial—in the living room. Nobody was watching. 'Jill?' I said. 'Peter?'

I wandered down the long hall, snapping on switches: Irene's sickroom, the upstairs bathroom, the master bedroom, Peter's domain. I did a double-take; he was there. Naked, lying on top of the bed, his still hand holding his penis—as if to keep it warm and safe—the head shining. The blades of the ceiling fan cut in slow circles above him. His eyes were vague and didn't turn my way; he was staring up. 'Oh sorry,' I whispered, 'God, sorry,' and flicked the light off again.

I headed back to the living room and sat, for a few seconds. When I'd collected myself, I went to find Jill. She wasn't in her downstairs room, which seemed typically adolescent in decor—Boy George poster, socks multiplying in a corner—until I spotted a quote from Rilke, in careful purple handwriting, taped for her long mirror: 'Beauty is only the first touch of terror we can still bear.'

I finally spotted the light under the basement bathroom door.

'Jill,' I said. 'It's me.'

'I'm in the bathroom,' she said.

'I know,' I said. 'I want to talk.'

She unlocked the door and let me in. She looked tense and peculiar; it looked as if she'd just thrown water on her face. She was still dressed in her clothes from the hospital—from the day before, the kelly-green sweat job—and she'd obviously been sitting on the edge of the tub, writing. There was a Papermate, a pad of yellow legal paper. The top sheet was covered with verses of tiny backward-slanting words. There was also last night's pot of Kraft Dinner on the sink. 'You're all locked in,' I said.

She didn't comment, and when the silence stretched on too long I said, 'Homework?' and pointed to the legal pad.

'No,' she said. Then she gave me a look and said, 'Poem.' 'Oh,' I said, and I was surprised. 'Do you ever show them? Or it?' 'No,' she said. 'They're not very good.' She sat back down on the tub. 'But maybe I'd show you, Aunt Adele.'

'Good,' I said. 'Not that I'm a judge.' I told her Irene was tucked in and that she was in a better, more positive frame of mind. More like herself. This seemed to relax Jill so much, I marched the lie a step further. 'Once your mum is out of the woods,' I said, 'your father may lighten up.' 'That day will never come,' she said.

'Never say never,' I said. I gave her a hug—she was so much bigger than my daughter, but I embraced her the same way I had Jane since she was born: a hand and a held kiss on the top of the head.

She hugged me back. 'Maybe I'll come live with you, Auntie A.' 'Maybe,' I said, mindful of Irene's wishes. 'You and everybody,' and saw the disappointment on her streaked face. So I added, 'Everything will be all right. Wait and see. She'll be all right.'

* * *

And Irene was. They claimed they'd got it, and ten days later she came home, earlier than expected. When Peter, Jill, and I were gathered around her in the sickroom, Irene started cracking jokes about her future prosthetic fitting. 'How about the Dolly Parton, hon?' she said to Peter. 'Then I'd be a handful.'

I was surprised to see Peter envelop her in his arm; I hadn't ever seen him offer an affectionate gesture. He told her he didn't care what size boob she bought, because breasts were for the hungry babies—not so much for the husband. I have these,' he said. 'These are mine. These big white shoulders.' And he rested his head against her shoulder and looked placidly at Jill; he was heavy, but Irene used her other arm to bolster herself, hold him up, and she closed her eyes in what seemed to be joy. Jill came and sat by me.

* * *

Irene took it easy the next few days; I stuck by, as did Jill, when she ventured in after school. I was shocked that there weren't more calls, or cards, or visitors except for Mum, and I realized my sister's life was actually very narrow, or extremely focused: family came first. Even Jill didn't seem to have any friends at all; the phone never rang for her.

Then Irene suddenly started to push herself—she prepared a complicated deep-fried Belgian dish; in the afternoon, she sat with Jill, in the Datsun, while Jill practiced parallel parking in front of the house and lobbied for a mother-daughter trip to lovely downtown Brooklyn for Christmas. And then, after a long nap and a little dinner, Irene insisted on attending the open house at Jill's school.

We were sitting listening to the band rehearse, a *Flashdance* medley, when I became aware of Irene's body heat—she was on my right—and asked if she might not want to head home. She was burning up. 'Let me get through this,' she said. Then Jill, on my other side, suddenly said in a small tight voice, 'Mum.' She was staring her mother's blouse, where a bright stitch of scarlet had shown up. Irene had bled through her dressing. Irene looked down. 'Oh,' she said. 'Peter.'

On the tear to the hospital, Peter said he'd sue Irene's stupid 'Paki bugger' doctor. He also said he should take his stupid wife to court for loss of sex. He should get a divorce for no-nookie. For supporting a one-tit wonder. And on and on.

Irene wasn't in shape to respond; I doubt she would have anyway.

Beside me in the back seat, Jill turned to stare out the window; she was white, sitting on her hands.

I found my voice. 'I don't think we need to hear this right now, Peter,' I said.

'Oh, Adele,' Irene said warningly. Disappointed.

He pulled over, smoothly, into a bus zone. Some of the people waiting for the bus weren't pleased. Peter turned and faced me, his finger punctuating. 'This is my wife, my daughter, my Datsun.' He paused. 'I can say what the hell I want. And you're welcome to walk.' He reached over and opened my door.

The two women at the bus shelter hurried away, correctly sensing an incident.

'I'm going with Aunt—' Jill was barely audible.

'No,' said Irene. 'You stay here.'

I sat there, paralyzed. I wanted to get out, but didn't want to leave Irene and Jill alone with him; Irene was very ill, Jill seemed defenceless. 'Look,' I said to Peter, 'forget I said anything. Let's just get Irene there, okay?'

He pulled the door shut, then turned front, checked me in the rearview one last time—cold, intimidating—and headed off again. Jill was crying silently. The insides of her glasses were smeared; I shifted over beside her and she linked her arm through mine tight, tight. Up front, Irene did not move.

* * *

They said it was an infection which had spread to the chest wall, requiring antibiotics and hospital admission. They were also going to perform more tests.

Peter took off with Jill, saying that they both had to get up in the morning.

Before I left Irene, she spoke to me privately, in a curtained cubicle in Emergency, and asked if I could stay at our mother's for the last few days of my visit; Irene didn't want to hurt me, but she thought it would be better, for all concerned, if I cleared out.

And then she went on; her fever was high, but she was lucid and fighting hard to stay that way. Could I keep quiet about this to our mother? And stop gushing about the East to Jill, going on about the Statue of Liberty and the view of the water from the window in the crown? And worry a little more about my own lost children and less about her daughter? And try to be more understanding of her husband, who sometimes wasn't able to exercise control over his emotions? Irene said Peter needed more love, more time; more of her, God willing. After that, she couldn't speak. And, frankly, neither could I.

I gave in to everything she asked. Jill and Peter dropped in together during the evening to see her; I visited Irene, with Mum, during the day when Peter was at work. Our conversations were banal and strained—they didn't seem to do either of us much good. After I left her one afternoon, I didn't know where I was going and ended up at my father's grave. I just sat there, on top of it, on the lap of the stone.

The day before my New York flight, I borrowed my mother's car to pick up a prescription for her at the mall. I was window-shopping my way back to the parking lot, when I saw somebody resembling my niece sitting on a bench outside a sporting goods store. At first, the girl seemed too dishevelled, too dirty-looking, actually, to be Jill, but as I approached, it became clear it was her. She wasn't doing anything. She sat there, draped in her mother's London Fog raincoat, her hands resting on her thickish thighs, clicking a barrette open, closed, open, closed. It was ten in the morning; she should have been at school. In English. For a moment, it crossed my mind that she might be on drugs: this was a relief; it would explain everything. But I didn't think she was. I was going to go over and simply say, *Yo, Jill, let's do tea*, and then I remembered my sister's frightening talk with me at the hospital and thought, *Fuck it. Butt out, Adele*, and walked the long way round. I turned my back.

* * *

One sultry Saturday morning, in late September—after I'd been back in Brooklyn for a few weeks—I was up on the roof preparing the first lessons for classes, when the super brought a handful of mail up. He'd been delivering it personally to tenants since the box had been ripped out of the entrance wall. It was the usual stuff and a thin white business envelope from Canada. From Jill. I opened it: *Dearlingest (sic) Aunt Adele, These are my only copies. Love, your only niece, Jill. P.S. I'm going to get a job and come see you at Easter.*

There were two. The poems were carefully written, each neat on their single page, with the script leaning left, as if blown by a stiff breeze. 'Black Milk' was about three deaths: before her beloved husband leaves for war, a nursing mother shares a bottle of old wine with him, saved from their wedding day, and unknowingly poisons her child and then herself. Dying, she rocks her dying child in her arms, but her last conscious thought is for her husband at the front. Jill had misspelled wedding; she'd put *weeding*.

'Belgium' described a young girl ice skating across a frozen lake—Jill had been to Belgium with her parents two times—fleeing an unnamed pursuer. During each quick, desperate glide, the ice melts beneath her until, at the end, she is underwater: 'In the deep cold / Face to face / Look, he comes now / My Father / My Maker.' The girl wakes up; it was a bad dream. And then her earthly father appears in her bed and, 'He makes night / Come again / All night,' by covering her eyes with his large, heavy hand.

I read these, and read them again, and I wept. I looked out, past the steeples and the tar roofs, where I thought I saw the heat rising, toward the green of Prospect Park, and held the poems in my lap, flat under my two hands. I didn't know what to do;

I didn't know what to do right away; I thought I should wait until I knew clearly what to say and whom to say it to.

* * *

In late October, Mum phoned, crying, and said that Irene's cancer had not been caught by the mastectomy. Stray cells had been detected in other areas of her body. Chemotherapy was advised. Irene had switched doctors; she was seeing a naturopath. She was paying big money for an American miracle gum, among other things.

Mum also said that Jill had disappeared for thirty-two hours. Irene claimed that Jill had been upset because of a grade—a C in Phys Ed. Mum didn't believe it was really that; she thought Irene's condition was disturbing Jill, but hadn't said that to Irene.

She didn't volunteer any information about the other member of Irene's family and I did not ask.

* * *

In November, Bill came east for a visit and brought the children, as scheduled; he also brought a woman named Cheryl Oak. The day before Thanksgiving, the two of them were invited to a dinner party, and I took Graham and Jane, taller and both painfully shy with me, to Central Park. It was a crisp, windy night. We watched the gi-normous balloons being blown up for the Macy's parade and bought roasted chestnuts, not to eat, but to warm the palms of our hands. I walked them back to their hotel and delivered them to the quiet, intelligent person who would probably become their stepmother, and be good to them, as she'd obviously been for Bill. Later, back in Brooklyn, I was still awake—wondering how another woman had succeeded with my husband and, now, my own little ones—when Irene phoned at 3 a.m. She told me Jill was dead. 'There's been an accident,' she said.

A few days later, my mother and stepfather picked me up at the Vancouver airport on a warm, cloudy morning. On the way to the funeral, they tried to tell me, between them—between breakdowns—what had happened. She had died of hypothermia; the impact of hitting the water had most likely rendered her unconscious. She probably hadn't been aware of drowning, but she'd done that, too. She'd driven the Datsun to Stanley Park—she'd told Irene she was going to the library—left the key in the ignition, walked not quite to the middle of the bridge, and hoisted herself over the railing. There was one eye-witness: a guy who worked in a video store. He'd kept saying, 'It was like a movie, I saw this little dumpling girl just throw herself off.'

The chapel was half-empty, and the director mumbled that that was unusual when a teenager passed on. Irene had not known, and neither had Mum, where to reach Joyce, our middle sister, who was missing as usual; Ray, our older brother, gave a short eulogy. He stated that he didn't believe in any God, but Irene did, and he was glad for that this day. He also guessed that when any child takes her own life, the whole family must wonder why, and probably do that forever. The face of my sister was not to be borne. Then we all sang 'The Water Is Wide', which Jill had once performed in an elementary-school talent show. She'd won Honourable Mention.

After the congregation dispersed, Peter remained on his knees, his head in his hands, while Irene approached the casket. Jill wore a pale pink dress and her other glasses, and her hair was pinned back, as usual, with a barrette—this time, a dove. Irene bent and kissed her on the mouth, on the forehead, then tugged at Jill's lace collar, adjusting it just so. It was the eternal mother's gesture, that finishing touch, before your daughter sails out the door on her big date.

I drank to excess at the reception; we all did, and needed to. Irene and I did not exchange a word; we just held each other for a long minute. From a distance, and that distance was necessary, I heard Peter talking about Belgium and memories of his childhood. On his fifth birthday, his sister, Kristin, had sent him a pencil from Paris, a new one, unsharpened, and he had used it until the lead was gone and it was so short he could barely hold it between his fingers. On the morning his mother was shot, in cold blood, he'd been dressing in the dark. The last thing she had said, to the Germans, was 'Don't hurt my little boy.' This was when Mum and I saw Irene go to him and take his hand. She led him down the hall to his bedroom and closed the door behind them. 'Thank God,' Mum said. 'Thank God, they have each other. Thank God, she has him.'

And for that moment, I forget about the despair that had prompted Jill to do what she did, and my own responsibility and silence, because I was alive and full of needs, sickness, and dreams myself. I thought, *No, I will never tell my sister what I suspect, because life is short and very hard*, and I thought, *Yes, a bad marriage is better than none*, and I thought, *Adele, let the sun go down on your anger, because it will not bring her back*, and I turned to my mother. 'Yes,' I said. 'Thank God.'

Source: "White Shoulders" reprinted from MARINE LIFE by Linda Svendsen. Copyright © 1982 by Linda Svendsen. Published by HarperCollins Publishers, Ltd. Reprinted by permission of the Author and Robin Straus Agency, Inc., New York.

Model APA Citation:

Svendsen, L. (1995). White shoulders. In M. Atwood & R. Weaver (Eds.), *The Oxford book of Canadian short stories in English* (pp. 413–422). Toronto: Oxford University Press. (Original work published 1992)

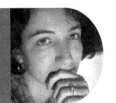

Discussion Questions:

1. According to Adele, the narrator of the story and Irene's sister, how has cancer physically affected Irene?

2. How does her Irene's cancer appear to affect Jill?

3. How does Irene's cancer appear to affect Peter?

4. What do you think is meant by Jill's statement when she is first told about her mother's cancer: "Don't die on me, Mum, or I'll kill you"?

5. What does Irene appear to be most concerned about throughout her illness?

6. Do Peter's various expressions of anger toward Irene surprise you? Why or why not?

7. What is ironic about the following line from the story: "Irene said Peter needed more love, more time; more of her, God willing."

8. What do Jill's poems suggest about her state of mind at the time of her suicide?

9. In the last paragraph of the story, Adele states "No. I will never tell my sister what I suspect…." What exactly is it that Adele suspects?

10. Do you think Svendsen's portrayal of how illness can damage a family is realistic? Why or why not?

11. Have you, or someone you are close to, ever been affected by a serious illness? How did you and/or your loved one cope?

12. What advice or support would you offer a family trying to cope with a difficult situation like the one in "White Shoulders"?

OTHER STORIES FOR YOUR CONSIDERATION

• "Cathedral" by Raymond Carver

A man initially hostile toward a blind man is transformed by his interaction with him.

Themes: blindness, disability, ignorance, discrimination

Model APA Citation:

Carver, R. (2008). Cathedral. In R.S. Gwynn & W. Campbell (Eds.), *Fiction: A pocket anthology* (2nd Can. ed., pp. 238–252). Toronto: Pearson. (Original work published 1983)

• "The Model" by Bernard Malamud

An aging man tries to ease his loneliness and recapture his youth by painting a young model.

Themes: aging, loneliness, alienation, reminiscence

Model APA citation:

Malamud, B. (1995). The model. In S. Marcus (Ed.), *A world of fiction: Twenty timeless short stories* (pp. 145–149). New York: Addison-Wesley. (Original work published 1983)

- "The Yellow Wallpaper" by Charlotte Perkins Gilman

A misunderstood woman mentally "unravels" in 19th century America.

Themes: mental illness, misdiagnosis, depression, confinement, insanity, repression

Model APA Citation:

Gilman, C.P. (2005). The yellow wallpaper. In R. S. Gwynn (Ed.), *Fiction: A pocket anthology* (4th

ed., pp. 88–103). New York: Pearson. (Original work published 1892)

- "Miss Brill" by Katherine Mansfield

A weekly ritual forces an aging woman to confront the harsh reality of her age and situation.

Themes: aging, ageism, isolation, reminiscence

Model APA Citation:

Mansfield, K. (2008). Miss Brill. In R.S. Gwynn & W. Campbell (Eds.), *Fiction: A pocket anthology*

(2nd Can. ed., pp. 119–123). Toronto: Pearson. (Original work published 1922)

- "The Use of Force" by William Carlos Williams

A power struggle ensues between a doctor and his child patient as he tries to diagnose her.

Themes: doctor–patient relationships, empathy, control

Model APA Citation:

Williams, W.C. (1952). *The use of force.* Retrieved from Classic Short Stories website: http://www.

classicshorts.com/stories/force.html

TRY IT YOURSELF

Using the previous model APA citations as a guide, for each of the remaining stories create your own APA reference page citation. Make sure to follow all APA rules regarding punctuation, capitalization, and italics. You will have to go to the library or use the Internet to locate the required information for each entry. Answers will vary so check with your instructor.

- "A Face of Stone" by William Carlos Williams

A doctor initially annoyed by two of his immigrant patients learns valuable lessons about judgment, courage, and survival.

Themes: doctor–patient relationships, prejudice, medical stress

Reference

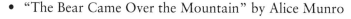

- "Good Country People" by Flannery O'Connor

A young lady with a wooden leg is taken advantage of by a smooth-talking bible salesman.

Themes: disability, alienation, difference, anger

Reference

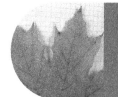

- "The Bear Came Over the Mountain" by Alice Munro

Alzheimer's disease impacts the life of a long-time married couple when the woman has to be institutionalized.

Themes: dementia, memory, loss, regret, reminiscence, fidelity, guilt, nursing homes

Reference

- "God is Not a Fish Inspector" by W. D. Valgaardson

A feisty elderly man hangs onto his pride and dignity despite various forces which work against him.

Themes: aging, inheritance, pride, reminiscence, nursing homes

Reference

- "A Rose For Emily" by William Faulkner

Emily Grierson is an eccentric and reclusive woman who mourns the loss of her lover in a very unusual way.

Themes: death, grief, mourning, madness

Reference

___

___

POEMS TO EXAMINE AND EXPLORE

The following two poems, "Do Not Go Gentle into That Good Night" (1952) by Dylan Thomas and "The Last Words of My English Grandmother" (1924) by William Carlos Williams, both explore the themes of death and dying. Thomas's poem is a plea from a son to his dying father to fight against his inevitable death, while Williams's poem portrays an elderly woman's fear and stubbornness as she is taken to the hospital in an ambulance. Read each poem carefully, and then work in small groups to discuss the questions that follow each reading.

DO NOT GO GENTLE INTO THAT GOOD NIGHT
by Dylan Thomas

Do not go gentle into that good night,
Old age should burn and rage at close of day;
Rage, rage against the dying of the light.

Though wise men at their end know dark is right,
Because their words had forked no lightning they
Do not go gentle into that good night.

Good men, the last wave by, crying how bright
Their frail deeds might have danced in a green bay,
Rage, rage against the dying of the light.

Wild men who caught and sang the sun in flight,
And learn, too late, they grieved it on its way,
Do not go gentle into that good night.

Grave men, near death, who see with blinding sight
Blind eyes could blaze like meteors and be gay,
Rage, rage against the dying of the light.

And you, my father, there on the sad height,
Curse, bless me now with your fierce tears, I pray.
Do not go gentle into that good night.
Rage, rage against the dying of the light.

Model APA Citation:

Thomas, D. (2009). Do not go gentle into that good night. In R. S. Gwynn (Ed.), *Literature: a pocket anthology* (4th ed., p. 643). New York: Pearson. (Original work published 1952)

Discussion Questions:

1. What repeated words and phrases do you notice in this poem? Make a list. Why do you think the poet chooses to repeat these words and phrases?

2. The word *death appears* only once in this poem. What are some of the indirect ways that the poet refers to death? Why do you think he chooses these phrases, rather than write about death directly?

3. Why do you think the speaker does not want his father to accept his death? Why does he ask him to fight? Would you ask the same of a loved one? Why or why not?

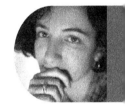

THE LAST WORDS OF MY ENGLISH GRANDMOTHER
by William Carlos Williams

There were some dirty plates
and a glass of milk

beside her small table
near the rank, dishevelled bed—

Wrinkled and nearly blind
she lay and snored
rousing with anger in her tones
to cry for food,

Gimme something to eat—
They're starving me—
I'm all right I won't go
to the hospital. No, no, no
you can do as you please.
She smiled, Yes
you do what you please first
then I can do what I please—

Oh, oh, oh! she cried
as the ambulance men lifted
her to the stretcher—
Is this what you call

making me comfortable?
By now her mind was clear—
Oh you think you're smart
you young people,

she said, but I'll tell you
you don't know anything.
Then we started.
On the way

we passed a long row
of elms. She looked at them
awhile out of
the ambulance window and said,

What are all those
fuzzy-looking things out there?
Trees? Well, I'm tired
of them and rolled her head away.

Model APA Citation:

Williams, W.C. (1941). The last words of my English grandmother. Retrieved from American Poems

website: http://www.americanpoems.com/poets/williams/9079

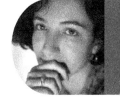

Discussion Questions:

1. What words would you use to describe the poet's grandmother's attitude and behaviour? Why do you think she behaves this way?

2. She says that she doesn't want to go to the hospital; why is she taken there in spite of her protests?

3. Have you experienced the aging, dementia, and/or death of a loved one? How did that person cope with the process?

4. What are the grandmother's last words? What do you think she means by them? What can readers learn from them?

OTHER POEMS FOR YOUR CONSIDERATION

- "When I have fears" by John Keats

Model APA Citation:

Keats. J. (2006). When I have fears. In J.S. Scot, R.E. Jones, & R. Bowers (Eds.), *The Harbrace anthology of literature* (4th ed., p. 145). Toronto: Nelson. (Original work published 1848)

- "King Lear in Respite Care" by Margaret Atwood

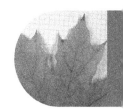

Model APA Citation:

Atwood, M. (1995). King Lear in respite care. Retrieved from The Poetry Archive website: http://
www.poetryarchive.org/poetryarchive/singlePoem.do?poemId=99

TRY IT YOURSELF

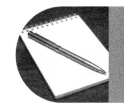

Using the previous model APA citations as a guide, for each of the remaining poems create your own APA reference page citation. Make sure to follow all APA rules regarding punctuation, capitalization, and italics. You will have to go to the library or use the Internet to locate the required information for each entry. As answers will vary, check with your instructor.

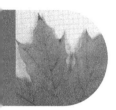

- "My Cancer Cure" by Robert Service

Reference

_____

_____

- "Waking in the Blue" by Robert Lowell

Reference

_____

_____

- "Tubes" by Donald Hall

Reference

_____

_____

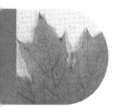

- "Five Days in the Hospital" by Alden Nowlan

Reference

_____

_____

- "In the Operating Room" by Alden Nowlan

Reference

_____

_____

FILMS TO WATCH AND INTERPRET

The following ten films are thematically related to health care. Your instructor may choose to show one or more in class, or you may opt to view some of them on your own or with classmates. Each film raises complex ethical issues that provide many points for you to discuss. For example, what ethical issues are involved in the

Fitzgeralds' decision to engineer a child to be a genetic match and donor for their first child, who has leukemia, in *My Sister's Keeper*? Or in John Nash's decision to stop taking his antipsychotic medication in *A Beautiful Mind*? Many of these films portray exemplary health care professionals, such as the title character in *Patch Adams* or Nurse Susie Monahan in *Wit*, while many others show health care professionals behaving unprofessionally or unethically, such as Nurse Ratched in *One Flew Over the Cuckoo's Nest* or Frank Pierce in *Bringing Out the Dead*. While watching these films, ask yourself how you would behave—as a patient, as a family member, as a health professional—in the situations depicted.

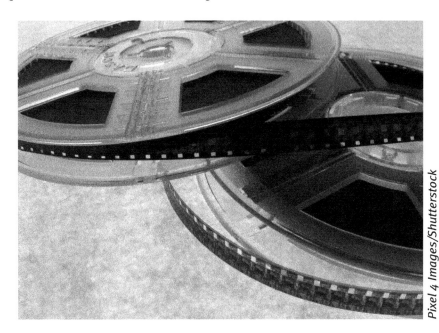

Pixel 4 Images/Shutterstock

- A Beautiful Mind (2001)

This Academy Award-winning film is based on the life of Nobel Prize-winning mathematician John Nash, who suffered from paranoid schizophrenia. As Nash witnesses the pain that his condition brings to his wife and friends, he also struggles with the decision to control his delusions through medication, knowing that it would impede his genius for mathematics, as well as his ability to connect emotionally to his wife.

Themes: schizophrenia, medication, delusions, genius, psychosis, paranoia

Model APA Citation:

Howard, R. (Director). (2002). *A beautiful mind*. [Motion picture]. United States: Universal Pictures.

- Bringing Out the Dead (1999)

Frank Pierce is a paramedic on the night shift in New York City, who is beginning to feel powerless to save lives. Collapsing under the burden of other people's pain and suffering, and unable to sleep, he repeatedly attempts to get fired.

Themes: paramedics, working with others, loss of patients, job burnout

Model APA Citation:

Scorsese, M. (Director). (1999). *Bringing out the dead.* [Motion picture]. United States: De Fina-Cappa.

- God Said "Ha!" (1998)

In a filmed monologue, comedian Julia Sweeney tells of caring for her brother Mike during the year between his cancer diagnosis and his death. First Mike and then her parents move in with her, and they use humour to cope with a tragic situation.

Themes: cancer, medical treatments, family support, humour, health insurance

Model APA Citation:

Sweeney, J. (Director). (1998). *God said "ha!"* [Motion picture]. United States: Oh Brother Productions Inc.

TRY IT YOURSELF

Using the previous model APA citations as a guide, for each of the remaining films create your own APA reference page citation. Make sure to follow all APA rules regarding punctuation, capitalization and italics. You will have to go to the library or use the Internet to locate the required information for each entry. As answers will vary, check with your instructor.

- My Sister's Keeper (2009)

This film, based on the book by Jodi Picoult, centres around a family trying to do everything they can to save their daughter from leukemia, including having a child by in vitro fertilization in order to supply genetic material to their dying daughter. The second daughter eventually rebels from her role as genetic donor and attempts to sue her parents.

Themes: bioethics, leukemia, autonomy, right to life, organ donation

Reference

_____

_____

- One Flew Over the Cuckoo's Nest (1975)

This classic multi-award winning film takes place mainly in a psychiatric ward. Convicted of statutory rape, Randle McMurphy pretends to be insane to avoid prison, and leads his fellow patients in a rebellion against the rigid routines and sterile environment of the psychiatric ward.

Themes: mental illness, mental health institutions, patient rebellion, depression, euthanasia, suicide, sanity, insanity, electroshock, lobotomy, power, control, abuse

Reference

_____

_____

- Patch Adams (1998)

This film is based on the true story of Hunter Adams, a man who is inspired to be a doctor for all the right reasons. His unusual approach to doctoring and healing draws both praise and criticism.

Themes: eccentricity, alternative healing methods, depression, doctor–patient relationships, rebellion, malpractice

Reference

_____

_____

- Sicko (2007)

The acclaimed documentary filmmaker Michael Moore sheds light on some of the failings of American health care by comparing it to systems in Canada, France, and Britain. Moore's documentary exposes some surprising injustices.

Themes: public health care, private health care, health insurance, quality of care, cost of care

_____

_____

- Vera Drake (2004)

Vera Drake is a character who takes medicine into her own hands in 1950s England by conducting abortions on women despite not being qualified to do so. Her illegal doctoring is eventually exposed and consequences follow.

Themes: abortion, ethics, nursing, malpractice

_____

_____

- What's Eating Gilbert Grape? (1993)

The Grape family consists of a single mother, who is both obese and agoraphobic, trying to raise her children, including her youngest who is autistic. This film explores some of the challenges faced by families dealing with mental illness and disability.

Themes: obesity, autism, depression, agoraphobia

_____

_____

- Wit (2001)

This film, based on the Pulitzer Prize-winning play by Margaret Edson, follows English professor Vivian Bearing as she undergoes experimental treatments for ovarian cancer. Vivian attempts to maintain her dignity and humanity as she realizes that her doctors see her as a research subject rather than a human being.

Themes: death and dying, doctor–patient relationships, nursing, experimental treatments, re-evaluation of values

_____

_____

INDEX